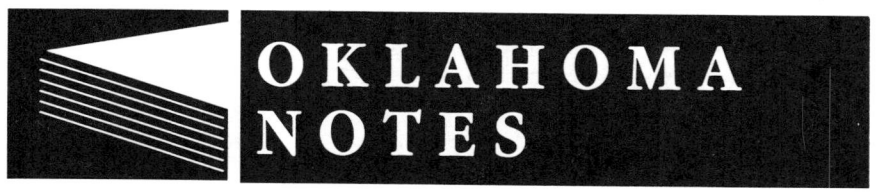

OKLAHOMA NOTES

Clinical Sciences Review for Medical Licensure
Developed at
The University of Oklahoma College of Medicine

Ronald S. Krug, *Series Editor*

Suitable Review for:
United States Medical Licensing Examination
(USMLE), Step 2

Springer
New York
Berlin
Heidelberg
Barcelona
Budapest
Hong Kong
London
Milan
Paris
Santa Clara
Singapore
Tokyo

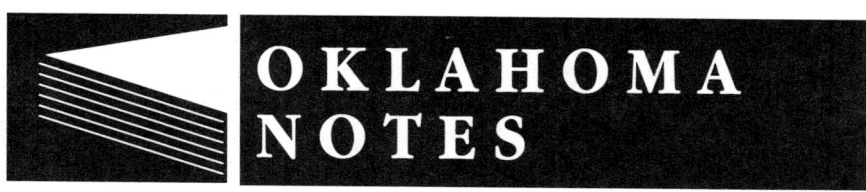

OKLAHOMA NOTES

Pediatrics

Second Edition

Edited by
Jane E. Puls
A. Eugene Osburn

Rita R. Claudet
Technical Editor

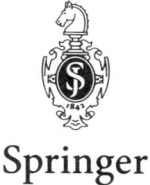

Springer

Jane E. Puls, M.D.
Department of Pediatrics
University of Oklahoma College of Medicine
Oklahoma City, OK 73190
USA

A. Eugene Osburn, D.O.
Department of Pediatrics
The University of Oklahoma College of Medicine,
Health Sciences Center
Oklahoma City, OK 73190
USA

Library of Congress Cataloging-in-Publication Data
Pediatrics / edited by Jane E. Puls, A. Eugene Osburn. — 2nd ed.
    p.   cm. — (Oklahoma notes)
    Includes bibliographical references.
    ISBN 0-387-94634-9
    1. Pediatrics—Outlines, syllabi, etc. I. Puls, Jane E.
II. Osburn, A. Eugene. III. Series.
    [DNLM: 1. Pediatrics—outlines. 2. Pediatrics—examination
questions. WS 18.2 P3707 1996]
RJ48.3.P44 1996b
618.92′0002′02—dc20
DNLM/DLC
for Library of Congress   96-13501

Printed on acid-free paper.

Production managed by Robert Wexler; manufacturing supervised by Joe Quatela.
Camera-ready copy prepared by the author.
Printed and bound by Edwards Brothers, Inc., Ann Arbor, MI.
Printed in the United States of America.

9 8 7 6 5 4 3 2 1

ISBN 0-387-94634-9 Springer-Verlag New York Berlin Heidelberg SPIN 10522818

Preface to the Oklahoma Notes

The intent of the Oklahoma Notes is to provide students with a set of texts that present the basic information of the general medical school curriculum in such a manner that the content is clear, concise and can be readily absorbed.

The basic outline format that has made the Oklahoma Notes extremely popular when preparing for standardized examinations has been retained in all the texts. The educational goals for these materials are first to help organize thinking about given categories of information, and second, to present the information in a format that assists in learning. The information that students retain best is that which has been repeated often, and has been actively recalled. The outline format has always been used in the Oklahoma Notes because students have reported to us that it allows them to cover subsequent parts of the outline, and use the topic heading as a trigger to recall the information under the heading. They then can uncover the material and ascertain whether they have recalled the information correctly.

This second edition of the Clinical Series of the Oklahoma Notes represents a major refinement of the first editions. A number of issues have been addressed to make the texts more efficient, effective and "user friendly." These include:

- Correction of technical errors.
- Addition of new material that has been reported since the first editions were published.
- Standard presentation of materials in all texts to make information more accessible to the student.
- Review questions written in standardized format. These questions reflect the major issues of the sections of the texts.

We hope these are helpful to you in your educational progress and preparation for required examinations.

Ronald S. Krug, Ph.D.
Series Editor

Preface

One learns medicine, including pediatrics, by first learning a set of rules and then spending the rest of his/her productive career discovering exceptions to those rules. This book is intended to serve as a study guide for organizing the acquisition of an initial foundation of information about pediatric topics. Without an initial set of rules all new information is simply another new rule, and not an interpretive frame of reference for the deeper level of understanding that occurs with the recognition that one is dealing with a change in his previously held belief. As such, we have attempted to include what we think most would agree are commonly held operational "facts" of pediatrics, and have not tried to justify or substantiate the facts with references or lengthy background information as to why these facts are currently thought to be true. Our primary intent in writing this book is to provide an adequate core of pediatric information to enable one to pass the pediatric portion of the national boards. We hope it will also provide a foundation for those who wish to spend more time discovering why children are different. If this study guide fulfills whichever of these needs is yours, it will have been successful.

Jane E. Puls, M.D.
A. Eugene Osburn, D.O.

Acknowledgments

No effort of this magnitude can be accomplished without a good deal of support. We could never have compiled our finished manuscript without the constant, late-night, do-whatever-it-takes help of our typist, Jody Chance. Her willingness to re-do and re-do and re-do resulted in a readable, formatted product that we hope addresses many pediatric issues. We appreciate her efforts and the unfailing support and help of Rita R. Claudet, MD, PhD, RS, our technical editor. Her constant enthusiasm and knowledge did much to lighten our load. The material in the chapters was willingly compiled by our contributors from their areas of expertise and interest, and we are grateful for their knowledge and ability to make pediatrics learnable and interesting. We also appreciate the input of Dr. Joan Parkhurst (Oncology) and Dr. Kent Ward (Cardiology), who helped us through some tricky areas. And we appreciate Rose Hayes, who always knows where we are and what we should be doing.

A great deal of our time and energy is in this book and our families know that time has been taken from them. They have tolerated (even encouraged) this with grace and good humor. To Harriet, Greg, Keri and Hilary (Dr. Osburn) and to Alan and infant Sarah (Dr. Puls), our deepest gratitude. All the evenings Sarah subsisted on animal crackers in the computer room at the hospital have surely been rewarded.

Contents

Contributors

Jill E. Adler, M.D., FAAP
Clinical Assistant Professor
Department of Pediatrics
University of Oklahoma
College of Medicine
Oklahoma City, Oklahoma

Jefry L. Biehler, M.D., MPH
Attending Physician
Miami Children's Hospital
Miami, Florida

Darin Brannan, M.D.
Instructor
Department of Pediatrics
University of Oklahoma
College of Medicine
Oklahoma City, Oklahoma

Peggy J. Hines, M.D., FAAP
Clinical Assistant Professor
Department of Pediatrics
University of Oklahoma
College of Medicine
Oklahoma City, Oklahoma

Veena Khanna, M.D., FAAP
Clinical Assistant Professor
Department of Pediatrics
University of Oklahoma
College of Medicine
Oklahoma City, Oklahoma

Diane Kittredge, M.D., FAAP
Associate Professor
Department of Pediatrics
University of Oklahoma
College of Medicine;
Director, Pediatric Practice Model
  for Continuity Care

Children's Hospital of Oklahoma
Oklahoma City, Oklahoma

Thomas A. Lera, II, M.D., FAAP
Associate Professor
Department of Pediatrics
University of Oklahoma
College of Medicine;
Medical Director
Children's Hospital of Oklahoma
Oklahoma City, Oklahoma

A. Eugene Osburn, D.O., FAAP, FACEP
Associate Professor
Department of Surgery
Director, Clinical Computing
Section of Emergency Medicine
University of Oklahoma
College of Medicine
Oklahoma City, Oklahoma

Jane E. Puls, M.D., FAAP
Assistant Professor
Department of Pediatrics
University of Oklahoma
College of Medicine
Oklahoma City, Oklahoma

Denise C. Scott, M.D., FAAP
Clinical Assistant Professor
Department of Pediatrics
University of Oklahoma
College of Medicine
Oklahoma City, Oklahoma

G. Edward Shissler, M.D., FAAP
Clinical Assistant Professor, Retired
Department of Pediatrics
University of Oklahoma
College of Medicine
Oklahoma City, Oklahoma

Morié Spencer, M.D., FAAP
Instructor
Department of Pediatrics
University of Oklahoma
College of Medicine
Oklahoma City, Oklahoma

Elias S. Srouji, M.D., MPH, FAAP
Professor
Department of Pediatrics
University of Oklahoma
College of Medicine
Oklahoma City, Oklahoma

Kendall L. Stanford, M.D., FAAP
Assistant Professor
Director, House Staff Recruitment
Director, House Staff Education
Department of Pediatrics
University of Oklahoma
College of Medicine
Oklahoma City, Oklahoma

Jill Stewart, M.D.
Instructor
Department of Pediatrics
University of Oklahoma
College of Medicine
Oklahoma City, Oklahoma

Roger Thompson, M.D.
Clinical Instructor
Department of Pediatrics
University of Oklahoma
College of Medicine
Oklahoma City, Oklahoma

Diane Kittredge
G Edward Shissler

The American Academy of Pediatrics (AAP) Committee on Practice and Ambulatory Medicine provides guidelines for a systematic approach to Health Maintenance Care which include the following components:

History
Physical Examination
Screening Procedures
         Growth Curve Measurements
             Height
             Weight
             Head Circumference
         Developmental Screening
         Cardiovascular Risk Screening
         Metabolic Screening
         Sensory Screening
         Hemoglobin/Hematocrit
         Urine Dipstick
         Tuberculin Test
         Lead Screening
Immunizations
Anticipatory Guidance and Health Education

Health Maintenance Care visits are scheduled to evaluate the child in each of the above areas. Details of the age-specific elements to be sought in each of these areas are found in numerous publications and practice protocols. The frequency of such visits is determined partially by the need to incorporate immunizations on a reasonable schedule, with additional visits scheduled to detect evolving problems as soon as practical. Listed in the tables below are highlights of such visits.

The medical history and physical examination are guided by anticipated problems for the age being evaluated, as well as by a Review of Systems and Complete Physical Exam to detect unanticipated problems.

Screening Procedures

Growth Screening

The height and weight should be plotted on age and sex appropriate growth curves at each visit. The head circumference should be measured and plotted for visits through age 18 months. Whether the child is following his/her curve is more important than any one individual measurement. Such growth curves are widely available. Below are methods for estimating expected growth parameters when such growth curves are not available.

The head circumference in term infants should grow at the following rate:
2 cm per month for the 1st three months
1 cm per month from 4-6 months
0.5 cm per month from 6-12 months

Height Estimation

Height	Centimeters	Inches
At birth	50	20
At 1 year	75	30
2-12 years	age (yr) x 6 + 77	age (yr) x 2.5 + 30

Body Weight Estimation

Age	Weight (kg)	
Newborn	3.5	Birth Weight (BW)
6 months	7	2 x BW
1 year	10	3 x BW
4 years	17.5	1/4 x AW
8 years	35	1/2 x AW
Adult	70	Adult Weight (AW)

Other growth parameters often useful to know are summarized in the following tables:

Surface Area Estimation Guidelines
$$SA\ (M^2) = [A \times Weight] + B$$

Weight (kg)	A	B
0 to 5	0.05	0.05
6 to 10	0.04	0.10
11 to 20	0.03	0.20
21 to 40	0.02	0.40

The anterior fontanel should close to palpation by 18 months of age. Some causes of a larger than normal or persistently open fontanel are:

Athyrotic hypothyroidism

Malnutrition

Progeria

Rubella syndrome

Russell-Silver syndrome

Hallermann-Streiff syndrome

Down syndrome

Trisomy 13 syndrome

Trisomy 18 syndrome

Alpert's syndrome

Kenny's syndrome

Aminopterin-induced syndrome

Achondroplasia

Pyknodysostosis

Vitamin D deficiency rickets

Osteogenesis imperfecta

Hypophosphatasia

Cleidocranial dysostosis

Expected Age of Deciduous Teeth Eruption

Tooth	Mean Age (months)	Age Range (months)
Lower central incisor	6	4 - 10
Upper central incisor	9	6 - 12
Upper lateral incisor	11.5	7 - 14
Lower lateral incisor	12	7 - 16
Upper first molar	15	12 - 18
Lower first molar	15.5	12 - 18
Lower cuspid	18	14 - 22
Upper cuspid	18	14 - 22
Lower second molar	26	22 - 30
Upper second molar	26	22 - 30

Developmental Screening

The child's developmental level should be assessed by history and examination at each visit. The Denver II is a widely used formal screening tool for ages 0 - 6 years. Below is a summary of highlights of developmental milestones for less formal use:

Age	Highlights of Developmental Milestones (Normal age range in months)	Developmental Warning Signs
2 weeks	**Lifts chin when prone** **Lies in flexed position** **Fixates to close objects and light**	Femoral click or hip instability (through 12 months) Undue maternal anxiety (true for all ages)
2 months	**Smiles** **Squeals** **Follows objects with eyes past midline**	Persistent heart murmur Absent response to noise Failure to fix gaze on face
4 months	**Lifts head and chest from prone** **Smiles at others (1.5-4)** **Rolls over front to back** **Follows objects with eyes 180 degrees** **Grasps rattle** **Coos and says "ah"**	Lack of bonding (a concern at any age)
6 months	**Sits without support (5-8)** **Transfers objects hand to hand (4.5-7)** **Babbles**	Failure to follow objects 180 degrees Persistent fisting Strabismus

9 months	Bears weight Crawls Pincer grasp (8.5-12) Uncover hidden toy Says nonspecific "Mama-Dada" Cruises holding furniture	Nystagmus Absence of babble Unable to sit alone
12 months	Stands alone (10-14) Says "Mama " or" Dada" (9-13) Walks well (11-15) Three words in addition to "Mama"	Unable to transfer objects hand to hand Absence of weight bearing while held
15 months	Walks backwards (12.5-21.5) Eats with a spoon	Unable to pull self to stand Abnormal grasp or pincer grip
18 months	Walks up steps (14-22) Finds hidden object (14-20) Stacks four cubes (15-20) Puts three words together	Open anterior fontanel Inability to walk alone Absence of constructive play Lack of spontaneous vocalization
24 months	Pedals tricycle (21-28) Combines 2 words (14-24) Kicks a ball forward on request	Absence of recognizable words

3 years	Uses plurals (21-36) **Balances on one foot (30-44)** **Goes up stairs** **Knows age** **Counts three objects**	Speech unintelligible to strangers
Preschool 3-6 years	**Stands 10 seconds on one foot by 5 years** **By school age, knows colors, counts to 10, hops on one foot, can heel-toe walk and speaks sentences of at least 10 syllables.**	Inability to perform self-care tasks: handwashing, simple dressing, daytime toilet
School age 6-12 years	**Is able to take formal tests to assess developmental level of achievement** **Sexual maturation begins around** **10 years in girls and 12 years in boys**	School failure Aggressive behavior such as firesetting
Adolescence	**Formal assessment tools can be used** **to quantitate level of functioning.**	School absenteeism or school failure

Cardiovascular Risk Screening

Blood pressure is measured routinely for children > 3 years of age. Blood lipid screening is done after 2 years of age if relevant family history and for all 18 year olds.

Metabolic Screening

The newborn is screened for hypothyroidism and the hyperphenylalaninemias including phenylketonuria (PKU) after 24 hours of age to insure an adequate protein intake for valid results. Infants discharged early may require a repeat screening at 2 weeks of age. More than 80% of states now also screen for hemoglobinopathies (which are more common than PKU or hypothyroidism). Other metabolic screening is dictated by family history and clinical suspicion. Some states routinely screen for a wide battery of metabolic disorders.

Sensory Screening

Hearing and vision are screened by subjective historical information and physical examination at each visit. Formal testing should be done before entering school, if not sooner because of a suspicious history or exam finding.

Hemoglobin/Hematocrit

Low-risk children fed iron-fortified formula for at least 9 months should be screened at 24 months, once in the school years, and at least once after puberty. Earlier and more frequent screening is indicated if risk factors exist.

Urinalysis

A urine dipstick for protein, blood and indications of infection (nitrate, leukocyte estrase) is recommended at least once in the preschool or school age period. Urinalysis and cultures are done if indicated by history or exam.

Tuberculin Test

The AAP and Centers for Disease Control and Prevention (CDC) recommend annual testing for children in high-risk populations (exposed to higher rates of TB than the USA national average or at medical risk for TB). Routine testing for low-risk groups is optional: at 12-15 months, school entry and once in adolescence.

Lead Screening

Screen low-risk children at 12 and 24 months; earlier and more frequent screening is indicated if the child lives or visits in a high-risk environment.

Routine Childhood Immunization

The list of effective vaccines and, secondarily, recommended immunization practice have changed rapidly during the last decade and can be expected to change even more rapidly in the next decade.

The following is an overview of routine childhood immunization. There is much more than this to learn; ie, about characteristics of vaccine-preventable diseases, about recognizing and reporting adverse events after vaccination, about contraindications and relative contraindications, about passive vs. active immunization, about vaccines not routinely given to children, etc.

Keeping Up

Your indispensable sources of information are the Committee on Infectious Diseases of the AAP and the Advisory Committee on Immunization Practices (ACIP) of the USPHS.

- The AAP *Red Book* is revised about every three years.
- Interim reports of the AAP Committee on Infectious Diseases are Published in *Pediatrics*, the Journal of the AAP.
- The ACIP publishes in the CDC's *Morbidity and Mortality Weekly Report (MMWR)*.

Types of Vaccine

- Live, attenuated viral vaccines (measles, mumps and rubella (MMR), varicella, and type 1, type 2, and type 3 polio (OPV)). These vaccines induce immunity by causing an actual infection, much milder than the natural disease.
- Toxoids (tetanus and diphtheria). These induce immunity to toxins generated by the organisms, but no immunity to the infection itself (without the toxin, the infection is benign).
- Vaccines consisting of fragments of organisms (hepatitis B (HB), *Haemophilus influenzae* (Hib), and the acellular pertussis in DTaP). The trick here is to find and use the fragment that will induce protective antibodies.
- Recombinant vaccine (HB). One of the HB vaccines is obtained from cultures of a recombinant yeast containing a portion of the gene that codes for an immunogenic bit of viral protein, hepatitis B surface antigen (HBsAg).
- Conjugated vaccines (Hib). Children under 2 years of age respond poorly to carbohydrate antigens; when the immunogenic antigen is a carbohydrate a much better response is attained if it is conjugated with a highly reactive protein.
- Killed whole organisms (pertussis). This is the one of the routine vaccines that causes the most side effects: it will probably be replaced entirely by a cell-fragment vaccine in the near future.

Recommended Schedule

Table I, endorsed by the AAP, the ACIP, and the American Academy of Family Practice, was published in January 1995. The varicella vaccine was added, at 12 to 18 months, in May 1995.

*   *Note:* Other looming changes include the use of DTaP instead of DTP for all vaccinations, and the use of IPV in the place of OPV at two and four months of age (an attempt to avoid the 8-9 cases of vaccine-induced polio seen each year in the USA).

A well-immunized 1 year old child will have received 10 or 11 injections (HB x 2 or 3, IPV x 2, diphtheria-tetanus-pertussis (DTaP) x 3, and Hib x 3), plus possibly one dose of trivalent OPV. By 2 years of age s/he will have received 15 injections (HB x 3, IPV x 2, DTaP x 4, Hib x 4, MMR, and varicella), plus 1 dose of OPV.

It is anticipated that over the next few years the number of injections will decrease as new combinations of vaccines are proven effective and are worked into the schedule (DTP and Hib are now available as a quadrivalent vaccine).

Age/Interval Minimums

Table II is taken from the CDC; General Recommendations on Immunization, *MMWR* 1994; 43: 1-38. It lists the minimum ages acceptable in the USA for administration of the routine childhood vaccines and the minimum acceptable intervals between doses. References in the footnotes are to other parts of the original publication.

Practitioners apply these minima daily as they review records of immunizations given outside their own practice, especially those given in other countries, where standard practices might be very different because of the local epidemiology of vaccine-preventable diseases and/or because of unavailability of medical services. Also, there will be times when a practitioner wants to use an accelerated immunization schedule (ie, when a patient will move soon to a medically underserved country, or when there is an opportunity to vaccinate a child who is underimmunized because of a family's medical noncompliance).

Contraindications

Absolute and permanent contraindications are rare:

- A severe allergic reaction to a previous dose of the vaccine in question or to one of its active or inactive ingredients (eg: anaphylactic reaction to neomycin would contraindicate MMR and IPV, to streptomycin, IPV).
- In the case of pertussis vaccine, the onset of encephalopathy within 7 days after a dose is given.

Contraindications that are relative and/or temporary include:

- Severe illness (vaccine side effects might make ongoing evaluation and management of the disease more difficult). Applies to all vaccines.
- Pregnancy (live vaccines are generally not given because theoretically there is risk to the fetus, but actual fetal injury has never been described). Applies only to live vaccines.
- Immunosuppression in the patient or, in the case of oral polio, in household contacts of the patient. Applies to live vaccines only.
  - *Note:* Currently infants who are HIV positive or who have AIDS should receive IPV instead of OPV and should receive the MMR. (ACIP makes this recommendation based on the high mortality from measles in children with AIDS, and the fact that there are no documented cases of vaccine-induced disease.)
- Recent receipt of blood products (antibodies in the blood product might prevent replication of the vaccine organism). Applies to live vaccines only.

A Recommended Approach to the Immunization of Children

An unacceptably large number of children in the USA are inadequately immunized, partly because health care providers have not placed enough emphasis on immunization. **If a health care provider sees a child and the child is eligible for immunization, the vaccine(s) should be given regardless of the primary purpose of the visit.**

TABLE I. **Recommended childhood immunization schedule*--United States, January 1995**

Vaccine	Birth	2 Months	4 Months	6 Months	12† Months	15 Months	18 Months	4 - 6 Years	11 - 12 Years	14 - 16 Years
Hepatitis B§	HB-1									
		HB-2		HB-3						
Diphtheria, Tetanus, Pertussis¶		DTP	DTP	DTP	DTP or DTaP at ≥ 15 months			DTP or DTaP	Td	
H. influenzae type b**		Hib	Hib	Hib	Hib					
Poliovirus		OPV	OPV	OPV				OPV		
Measles, Mumps, Rubella††				MMR				MMR or →	MMR	

* Recommended vaccines are listed under the routinely recommended ages. Shaded bars indicate range of acceptable ages for vaccination.

† Vaccines recommended in the second year of life (i.e., 12-15 months of age) may be given at either one or two visits.

§ Infants born to hepatitis B surface antigen (HBsAg)-negative mothers should receive the second dose of hepatitis B vaccine between 1 and 4 months of age, provided at least 1 month has elapsed since receipt of the first dose. The third dose is recommended between 6 and 18 months of age. Infants born to HBsAg-positive mothers should receive immunoprophylaxis for hepatitis B with 0.5 ml Hepatitis B Immune Globulin (HBIG) within 12 hours of birth, and 0.5 ml of either Merck Sharpe & Dohme (West Point, Pennsylvania) vaccine (Recombivax HB®) or SmithKline Beecham (Philadelphia) vaccine (Engerix-B®) at a separate site. In these infants, the second dose of vaccine is recommended at 1 month of age and the third dose at 6 months of age. All pregnant women should be screened for HBsAg during an early prenatal visit.

¶ The fourth dose of diphtheria and tetanus toxoids and pertussis vaccine (DTP) may be administered as early as 12 months of age, provided at least 6 months have elapsed since the third dose of DTP. Combined DTP-Hib products may be used when these two vaccines are administered simultaneously. Diphtheria and tetanus toxoids and acellular pertussis vaccine (DTaP) is licensed for use for the fourth and/or fifth dose of DTP in children aged ≥ 15 months and may be preferred for these doses in children in this age group.

** Three H. influenzae type b conjugate vaccines are available for use in infants: 1) oligosaccharide conjugate Hib vaccine (HbOC) (HibTITER®, manufactured by Praxis Biologics, Inc. [West Henrietta, New York], and distributed by Lederle-Praxis Biologicals, [Wayne, New Jersey]); 2) polyribosylribitol phosphate-tetanus toxoid conjugate (PRP-T) (Act HIB™, manufactured by Pasteur Mérieux Sérums & Vaccins, S.A. (Lyon, France), and distributed by Connaught Laboratories, Inc. [Swiftwater, Pennsylvania], and OmniHIB™, manufactured by Pasteur Mérieux Sérums & Vaccins, S.A., and distributed by SmithKline Beecham); and 3) Haemophilus b conjugate vaccine (Meningococcal Protein Conjugate) (PRP-OMP) (PedvaxHIB®, manufactured by Merck Sharp & Dohme). Children who have received PRP-OMP at 2 and 4 months of age do not require a dose at 6 months of age. After the primary infant Hib conjugate vaccine series is completed, any licensed Hib conjugate vaccine may be used as a booster dose at age 12-15 months.

†† The second dose of measles-mumps-rubella vaccine should be administered EITHER at 4-6 years of age OR at 11-12 years of age.

Source: Advisory Committee on Immunization Practices, American Academy of Pediatrics, and American Academy of Family Physicians.

Table II. Minimum age for initial vaccination and minimum interval between vaccine doses, by type of vaccine.[1] -- United States, 1994.

Vaccine	Minimum *age* for first dose*	Minimum *interval* from dose 1 to 2*	Minimum *interval* from dose 2 to 3*	Minimum *interval* from dose 3 to 4*
DTP (DT)[†]	6 weeks[§]	4 weeks	4 weeks	6 months
Combined DTP-Hib	6 weeks	1 month	1 month	6 months
DTaP*	15 months			6 months
Hib (primary series)				
HbOC	6 weeks	1 month	1 month	¶
PRP-T	6 weeks	1 month	1 month	¶
PRP-OMP	6 weeks	1 month	¶	
OPV	6 weeks[§]	6 weeks	6 weeks	
IPV**	6 weeks	4 weeks	6 months[††]	
MMR	12 months[§§]	1 month		
Hepatitis B	birth	1 month	2 months[¶]	

DTP -- Diphtheria-tetanus-pertussis	IPV -- Inactivated poliovirus vaccine
DTaP -- Diphtheria-tetanus-acellular-pertussis	MMR -- Measles-mumps-rubella
Hib -- Haemophilus influenzae type b conjugate	OPV -- Live oral polio vaccine

* These minimum acceptable ages and intervals may not correspond with the optimal recommended ages and intervals for vaccination.

[†] DTaP can be used in place of the fourth (and fifth) dose of DTP for children who are at least 15 months of age. Children who have received all four primary vaccination doses before their fourth birthday should receive a fifth dose of DTP (DT) or DTaP at 4-6 years of age before entering kindergarten or elementary school **and** at least 6 months after the fourth dose. The total number of doses of diphtheria and tetanus toxoids should not exceed six each before the seventh birthday (14).

[§] The American Academy of Pediatrics permits DTP and OPV to be administered as early as 4 weeks of age in areas with high endemicity and during outbreaks.

¶ The booster dose of Hib vaccine which is recommended following the primary vaccination series should be administered no earlier than 12 months of age **and** at least 2 months after the previous dose of Hib vaccine.

** See text to differentiate conventional inactivated poliovirus vaccine from enhanced-potency IPV.

[††] For unvaccinated adults at increased risk of exposure to poliovirus with <3 months but >2 months available before protection is needed, three doses of IPV should be administered at least 1 month apart.

[§§] Although the age for measles vaccination may be as young as 6 months in outbreak areas where cases are occurring in children <1 year of age, children initially vaccinated before the first birthday should be revaccinated at 12-15 months of age and an additional dose of vaccine should be administered at the time of school entry or according to local policy. Doses of MMR or other measles-containing vaccines should be separated by at least 1 month.

¶ This final dose is recommended no earlier than 4 months of age.

[1] Adapted from CDC. General Recommendations on Immunization. *MMWR* 1994; 43: 1-38.

Anticipatory Guidance and Health Education

This includes counseling and advice given in the following areas:

Child Development
Help parents understand and anticipate developmental milestones.
Advise activities to optimize developmental progress.

Child Behavior
Help parents understand and respond appropriately to normal stages of infant and child behaviors.
Guide parents in psychosocial aspects of child rearing (eg, child care, discipline).

Nutrition
Respond to concerns about feeding and mealtime behavior.
Offer counseling to improve nutrition and establish healthy eating habits for life.

Safety
Provide counseling about common injuries at each age period and recommend strategies to reduce risks.

Medical Concerns
Anticipate potential risks for dysfunction and diseases, and provide counseling and health education as indicated (eg, fluoride supplementation to reduce dental caries; anticipatory planning to provide optimal medical services for children with chronic diseases, etc.).

Leading Injury Deaths In USA, Ages 0-14 Years
1980-1985

Death rate/ 100,000/year		Etiology	Prevention
8.1	#1	Motor Vehicle Accident Occupant, Pedestrian and Bike related	Car seats < 4 years Seat belts > 4 years Street safety Helmets when biking, skating, etc.
2.8	#2	Drowning	Pool fences, life jackets, water safety and swimming lessons
2.3	#3	House fires	Smoke alarms Child proofing homes: cigarette lighters, matches, fuels, etc.
1.9	#4	Homicide	Child abuse prevention services, gun control, substance abuse services
0.7	#5	Suffocation and strangulation	Product regulation: cribs, plastic bags, pacifiers, toys, etc.
0.6	#6	Unintentional firearms	Guns unloaded and locked away

Common Safety Hazards by Age Group		
Age Range	**Hazard**	**Prevention**
Early Infancy	Crib safety Scald burns MVA injuries Rolling off high surface Foreign body aspiration	Slats less than 2 3/8 inches apart Water-heater temperature <120°F Car seats Do not leave unattended Keep small toys and objects out of reach
Late Infancy	Poisonous ingestions Increased mobility MVA injuries	Restrict access to poisonous substances Protect from open windows, electric cords, wall sockets, stairways and water hazards Forward facing car seat when >20 lbs
Pre-school	Unsafe use of toys or perceived toys Bites from "pets" Auto/Pedestrian accidents	Teach playground safety Do not allow access to guns, knives, etc. Teach appropriate respect for animals Teach traffic safety
School Age	Bicycle accidents Sports injuries Drowning	Bicycle helmets Protective equipment, supervised sports Water safety
Adolescence	Feelings of invulnerability	Education and support to lessen self and peer pressure induced vehicular, substance abuse, and sexually-transmitted injuries

Jill Adler

Developmental Considerations

The infant's intrauterine stay is divided into two periods: embryonic, which consists of the first 12 weeks post fertilization, and fetal, which refers to the remainder of intrauterine life. Organogenesis occurs in the first 12 weeks of embryonic development, following which the fetus experiences somatic growth and differentiation of organ systems. In the first half of the gestational period, development occurs by hyperplasia (an increase in the number of cells), and in the second half by hypertrophy (increase in cell size).

The fetus begins making respiratory efforts during the first half of gestation, but alveolar development sufficient to maintain extrauterine respiration does not occur until approximately 24 weeks gestation. Surfactant production (which aids in lung expansion and protects against atelectasis) is present as early as 20 weeks gestation, but adequate levels are usually not found until 35 weeks gestation. However, the fetus is generally considered to be viable at 24 to 26 weeks of gestation.

Growth of the fetus requires transfer of nutrients between the mother and infant. This function is carried out by the placenta, which also carries out the primary function of gas exchange. In addition, it produces hormones which support and regulate the pregnant state. Although the placenta demonstrates selectivity of substances transferred, it does not prevent passage of many bacteria, viruses and drugs. This accounts for many intrauterine and post-natal pathologic states of the infant, as does failure to provide for the metabolic needs of the infant.

The normal gestational period is 40 weeks (280 days from the first day of the last menstrual period) and infants born at less than 38 weeks gestation are considered pre-term. Infants born at greater than 42 weeks gestation are considered post-term.

During labor and birth, the greatest risk to the infant is from interruption of placental blood flow. This can occur with umbilical cord compression, which causes fetal hypoxia or with placental abruption, which causes both hypoxia and hypovolemia. Most traumatic effects of labor are of minor clinical significance. Occasionally, maternal anesthesia may cause depression of the infant. When the infant is born and begins respiratory efforts, dramatic changes in gas exchange occur.

Before birth, only 10-15% of fetal circulation perfuses the lungs. Oxygenated blood from the placenta flows to the right atrium via the inferior vena cava and then to both ventricles, because the foramen ovale is present. The left ventricle primarily perfuses the brain and myocardium, and the right ventricle perfuses the lower body via the ductus arteriosus. A state of relative right ventricular hypertrophy exists (pressures are approximately equal in the left and right sides of the circulatory system). After transition to extrauterine life, pulmonary blood flow increases 8 to 10 fold due to closure of the foramen ovale and ductus arteriosus. Blood flows from the right atrium to the right ventricle and then through the lungs (where it is oxygenated) via the pulmonary artery. The oxygenated blood is returned to the left atrium and ventricle for distribution to the systemic circulation via the aorta. Systemic blood returns to the right atrium via the vena cava. In the first 12 hours after birth functional closure of the ductus occurs and the circulatory flow pattern that will persist through life is completed.

Diagnostic Modalities

History
> Known heritable family disorders
> Maternal age
> Parity
> Date of last menstrual period
> Maternal drug use or smoking
> Maternal infections
> Prenatal care
> Maternal screening for diabetes, hepatitis, sickle cell disease (if appropriate)
> Labor
> > Onset and duration
> > Time of rupture of membranes
> > Intrapartum fetal distress
> > Type of delivery (vaginal, vacuum extraction, forceps, cesarean section)
> > Apgars

Physical Examination
> Vital signs
> Height, weight, FOC
> Determination of approximate gestational age (Dubowitz)
> Head - cephalhematoma, caput, scalp electrode, size of anterior and posterior fontanels, general shape
> Ears - shape, position, skin tags, ear canal patency
> Eyes - red reflex, opacification of lens (congenital cataract), shape
> Nares - patency
> Oropharynx - shape and integrity of soft and hard palates, sucking reflex
> Neck - presence or absence of clavicular fractures, lymphadenopathy
> Thorax - symmetry, presence or absence of retractions
> Cardiovascular - rate, presence or absence of murmur, gallop, thrill, character of peripheral pulses

Lungs - respiratory rate, equality of breath sounds, crackles, retractions

Abdomen - character of umbilicus, number of umbilical vessels, presence or absence of masses, organomegaly, bowel sounds, bilateral palpation of the kidneys

Genitalia - female: differentiation, presence or absence of clitoromegaly; male: presence or absence of hypospadias, presence or absence of testicles, hernia, hydrocele

Rectum - patency of anus

Skin - lanugo, vernix, dry, scaly skin, nevi

Neuro - presence or absence of grasp reflexes (palmar and plantar), sucking reflex, moro reflex

Laboratory Data

Coombs' determination in infants with mothers who are Rh- or O+ blood type

In infants who are small or large for gestational age polycythemia, hypocalcemia and/or hyper or hypoglycemia may occur, so determinations of hematocrit, calcium and serum glucose may be necessary.

Delivery Room Management

The need for resuscitation is assessed by use of the Apgar scoring system. It is routinely done at one minute and five minutes after birth. Usual scores are >5 at one minute and 8 or 9 by five minutes.

Apgar Score			
Score	**0**	**1**	**2**
Appearance	blue, pale	body pink, acrocyanosis	no cyanosis
Pulse	absent	< 100/minute	> 100/minute
Grimace	no response	grimace	sneeze or cough
Activity	flaccid	weak flexion	strong flexion
Respiratory effort	absent	weak, irregular	strong, regular

The infant is dried and provided necessary temperature support.

The eyes are protected from gonococcal ophthalmia with Silver nitrate or erythromycin ophthalmic ointment.

The infant is given intramuscular vitamin K to facilitate synthesis of coagulation factors.

A heel stick is done to measure the blood glucose level. A level below 30-40 mg/dl in the normal term infant is considered hypoglycemia for the first couple of hours after birth. Thereafter, a level below 40 mg/dl is abnormal.

As soon as is feasible, the infant is presented to the mother to initiate infant-maternal bonding.

Identification of risk factors or problems dictate additional measures as appropriate.

Neonatal Feeding

The initiation of feeding in the newborn is determined by the type of nutrition desired by the mother. Mothers who wish to breast feed may institute feeding as early as the delivery room in a normal, healthy term infant. For approximately 48 to 72 hours, the mother's breasts provide colostrum. Colostrum is produced in lower volume than breast milk, is higher in protein content and contains immunologic factors. It and breast milk are nutritionally complete foods for the newborn infant.

Breast feeding is not possible for many preterm infants, especially those in the neonatal intensive care unit who are intubated or too young to have an adequate suck. Mothers of preterm infants may express milk which can be fed to their infants by gavage or specially designed bottle and nipple.

Mothers who are HIV positive should not breast feed, as it is possible to infect the infant via viral particles present in breast milk.

If an infant's mother chooses to feed formula, the first feeding usually consists of sterile water. Thus, infants with tracheoesophageal fistula or neurological impairment of swallowing will hopefully demonstrate these abnormalities before a milk feeding, which is more irritating to lung tissue.

The average term infant will take 30 to 60 ml of formula every three hours the first few days of life, but feeding needs vary dramatically. The average infant requires 100-120 calories per kilogram per day for adequate growth. Infants generally lose weight the first 5 to 7 days of life. They should have regained this and be back to birth weight by approximately 14 days of life.

If an infant fails to demand adequate amounts of breast milk or formula at reasonable intervals, a variety of etiologies should be considered. Sepsis, metabolic abnormalities, transplacental passage of drugs used for pain control during delivery, magnesium given for maternal hypertension and central nervous system abnormalities should be considered as possible etiologies.

Neonatal Screening

Infants are routinely screened for hypothyroidism, PKU, galactosemia and sickle cell diseases in most states. Infants born at home or who are discharged early (within 24 hours) from the hospital after birth need to be followed closely by their primary physician and insure that adequate screening occurs.

Pathophysiologic Manifestations

Respiratory Distress in the Newborn

Respiratory distress is one of the most common problems encountered in the newborn infant. Although the most prominent physical abnormalities are in the respiratory system, the causes are myriad. The most important of these (starred) will be discussed in the Disease Profile section. Physical findings suggestive of respiratory distress include a sustained respiratory rate of over 60 per minute, nasal flaring, chest wall retractions, cyanosis, expiratory grunting or persistent cough.

Causes of Neonatal Respiratory Distress
Respiratory Disorders

Upper airway obstruction
Choana atresia
Vocal cord paralysis
Meconium aspiration
Transient tachypnea of the newborn
Pneumonia
★Hyaline Membrane Disease
Pneumothorax
Pleural effusions
Structural lung abnormalities

Cardiac Disorders

Left-sided outflow obstruction
Hypoplastic left heart
Aortic stenosis
Coarctation of the aorta
Cyanotic heart disease
Transposition of the great vessels
Total anomalous pulmonary venous return
Tricuspid atresia
Hypoplastic right heart
Right-sided outflow obstruction

Other Disorders
★Sepsis
Hypothermia
Hyperthermia
Hypoglycemia
Polycythemia
Metabolic acidosis
CNS lesions
Neuromuscular lesions
Phrenic nerve palsy
Diaphragmatic hernia

Neonatal Seizures

This is not a single disease entity: metabolic disorders, toxic exposures, sepsis/meningitis, hypoxemia, CNS hemorrhage and congenital CNS anomalies may all manifest with seizure activity. The neuronal development of the neonatal brain is incomplete, so that generalized tonic-clonic seizures are difficult to generate and are the least common variant.

Types of Neonatal Seizures
Focal - unilateral rhythmic movements most commonly localized to the face or extremities - associated with structural lesions, infection, subarachnoid hemorrhage
Myoclonic - brief jerking primarily of distal muscle groups (may be focal or generalized)
Tonic - rigid posturing of extremities and/or trunk; may also note eye deviation
Clonic - rhythmic motions of multiple muscle groups
Brief or subtle seizures may be demonstrated by lip smacking, tongue thrusting, blinking, bicycling of extremities, apnea and color changes

Since neonatal seizures may be subtle, diagnosis can be difficult. It is not unusual for these to be associated with tachycardia and hypertension. Seizure activity cannot be suppressed by restraint. Telemetric EEG monitoring may be useful.

Because the existence of seizures in the neonatal usually indicates significant organic disease, it is imperative to establish the etiology as early as possible.

The eyes should be examined for evidence of TORCH infection (chorioretinitis). The skin should be inspected for signs of neurocutaneous disorders (tuberous sclerosis, Sturge-Weber, neurofibromatosis). Serum electrolytes should be obtained to look for disturbances in glucose, calcium, magnesium and BUN.

A lumbar puncture should be performed and examined for signs of hemorrhage or infection.

If an inborn error of metabolism is suspected, evidence of metabolic acidosis or anion gap should be looked for. Serum ammonia, lactate, urine and serum organic acids may help identify the etiology.

If toxic exposure or maternal drug use are suspected a urine drug screen may identify the agent.

If CNS hemorrhage or structural abnormality are suspected, a CT scan or MRI should be obtained.

Disease Profiles

Hyaline Membrane Disease
Major cause of death in the newborn period. Occurs primarily in premature infants. Due to deficiency of pulmonary surfactant, reduced number of alveoli and increased chest wall compliance resulting in hypoxemia, hypercarbia and acidosis.

Alternate Terminology
Respiratory Distress Syndrome of the Newborn

Etiology
Absence or immature levels of pulmonary surfactant, which leads to alveolar atelectasis, hyaline membrane formation and interstitial edema.

Predisposing Conditions
Prematurity (especially if < 37 weeks gestation), infants of diabetic mothers, multiple gestation, cesarean section delivery, precipitous delivery, asphyxia, cold stress, family history of other affected infants.

Symptoms
Tachypnea, grunting, chest wall retractions, nasal flaring, cyanosis, apnea, irregular respirations

Physical Examination
Breath sounds may be normal or decreased; crackles may be heard with inspiration

Laboratory Findings
Respiratory acidosis or mixed respiratory/metabolic acidosis, hypoxemia

Differential Diagnosis
Group B streptococcal sepsis
Pneumonia

Cyanotic heart disease
Transient tachypnea of the newborn
Persistent fetal circulation

Potential Complications
Pneumothorax
Interventricular (cerebral) hemorrhage
Bronchopulmonary dysplasia
Retrolintylribroplasia (RLF) associated with the use of high levels of O_2

Diagnostic Plan
Diagnosis based on physical examination plus X-ray, measurement of arterial blood gases

Therapeutic Plan
Administration of artificial surfactant shortly after birth, administration of oxygen (frequently via mechanical ventilation), supportive care to reduce acidosis, hypotension and hypothermia

Neonatal Sepsis
The term sepsis refers to bacteremia in conjunction with some or all of the following: apnea, cyanosis, hypotension, disseminated intravascular coagulation. Neonatal sepsis may occur anytime in the first six months of life.

Alternate Terminology
Sepsis neonatorum

Etiology
Most common pathogens
Group B streptococcus
Escherichia coli
Listeria monocytogenes
Sites of entry for these organisms include breaches in the skin, umbilical cord, lungs, gastrointestinal tract and urinary tract.

Pathophysiology
Neonates may have relative or absolute deficiencies in their immune system due to decreased passive transplacental passage of maternal IgG. Neutrophil function may be impaired and relative granulocytopenia may occur.

Predisposing Conditions
Low birth weight
Maternal fever and/or leukocytosis during labor and delivery
Maternal chorioamnionitis
Prolonged rupture of membrane
Male sex
Twin birth

Congenital anomalies
Immune deficiency disorders
Galactosemia

Symptoms

Temperature instability
Poor feeding
Apnea
Tachypnea
Irritability

Physical Examination

Exam abnormalities related to affected organ(s)
Fever or hypothermia may be present
Hypotension
Cyanosis
Grunting, retractions and/or nasal flaring

Laboratory Findings

Positive blood culture (+/-)
Elevated total white blood count (or neutropenia)
Left shift on differential

Differential Diagnosis

Hyaline membrane disease
Hypothyroidism
Drug withdrawal
Congenital cardiac disease
Infections of single organ systems (meningitis, pneumonia, urinary tract infection)

Potential Complications

Mortality rate 10-70%. End organ dysfunction may occur with shock. Persistent fetal circulation.

Therapeutic Plan

If sepsis is **suspected**, appropriate cultures (blood, urine, CSF) should be obtained and treatment instituted **before** the diagnosis is confirmed. Newborns may deteriorate very rapidly and proceed to shock or death. Any early indication of sepsis must be acted on immediately. Ampicillin and gentamicin or cefotaxime is the antibiotic regimen of choice.

Hyperbilirubinemia

Almost 50 percent of all newborns develop clinical jaundice after birth (jaundice usually detectable with serum bilirubin of 7 mg/dl or greater). Approximately 8% of all newborns have a serum bilirubin greater than 15 mg/dl. Most neonatal jaundice is not considered pathologic.

Alternate Terminology
>Neonatal jaundice

Etiology
>Physiologic
>
>Nonphysiologic - common causes
>>Coombs' positive - Rh, ABO incompatibility
>>Coombs' negative
>>>Polycythemia
>>>Hepatitis
>>>Intrauterine infections
>>>Sepsis
>>>Galactosemia
>>>Spherocytosis
>>>Enclosed hemorrhage
>>>Infant of diabetic mother
>>>Premature infant
>>>Hypothyroidism

Pathophysiology

Bilirubin is produced primarily from the breakdown of red-cell hemoglobin. The enzyme bilirubin reductase reduces bilirubin to bilirubin IXa.

The newborn has a greater red cell mass than older individuals and its red cells have a 25 percent shorter life span. Most bilirubin is bound to available albumin and is transported to the liver for conjugation, which converts it to a water soluble form. After conjugation, bilirubin is excreted into the bile. The newborn liver is not an efficient conjugator of bilirubin. The presence of bacteria in the gut inhibits resorption of conjugated bilirubin, but the gut is sterile in the newborn, and bilirubin may be resorbed via the enterohepatic circulation.

All of the above cause increased levels of serum bilirubin in the newborn infant.

Physiologic jaundice is characterized by a healthy term infant, whose serum bilirubin rises to > 6 to 8 mg/dl on the third day of life and then falls to < 1.5 mg/dl by the tenth day of life.

Kernicterus is a disease characterized by the presence of marked jaundice (serum bilirubin usually > 25 mg/dl in term infants) with yellow staining of the brain, usually affecting the basal ganglia, globus pallidus, putamen and caudate nuclei. Initially infants also present with decreased tone, vomiting and/or poor feeding, and a high pitched cry. As the disease worsens, it may progress to seizures, fever, rigidity, opisthotonos and paralysis of upward gaze. Many affected infants die, but surviving children develop spasticity, athetosis, some degree of deafness, mental retardation and paralysis of upward gaze. Infants with Rh disease, ABO incompatibility and/or prematurity may be susceptible to kernicterus at lower levels of serum bilirubin (18-20 mg/dl). Kernicterus is now an uncommon disease.

Predisposing Conditions
Prematurity
Traumatic labor and/or delivery
Maternal illness during pregnancy (congenital viral infection or toxoplasmosis)
Maternal use of sulfonamides, nitrofurantoin, antimalarials (especially in family with G6PD family history)
Delayed cord clamping (polycythemia)
Maternal chorioamnionitis
Maternal diabetes
Infants small for gestational age (polycythemia, intrauterine infections)
Microcephaly (in utero infection)
Extravascular blood (cephalhematoma, extensive bruising)
Petechiae (congenital infection, sepsis, erythroblastosis)
Hepatosplenomegaly (congenital infections, hemolytic anemia, liver disease)

Symptoms
Clinical jaundice
Lethargy
Poor feeding
Or symptoms associated with specific disease predisposing to hyperbilirubinemia

Physical Examination
Scleral staining is first clinical sign
Jaundice frequently is noticeable next over the thorax and then is apparent on the face

Laboratory Findings
Total serum bilirubin is elevated. In physiologic jaundice the indirect bilirubin is disproportionately higher than the direct bilirubin.

If nonphysiologic jaundice is suspected, a Coombs' test should be obtained, as well as a serum hematocrit, reticulocyte count and examination of peripheral smear.

Positive Coombs' - Rh isoimmunization, ABO incompatibility or other antibody factors will be present.

High hematocrit - polycythemia

Low hematocrit - hemolysis, hemorrhage, red cell membrane defect most likely

Reticulocyte count abnormal - red cell membrane defect, ABO incompatibility, drugs, DIC

Differential Diagnosis

Once hyperbilirubinemia is established, the differential is as above.

Potential Complications

Kernicterus

Death

Therapeutic Plan

In term infants, with serum bilirubin peaking at 20 mg/dl on day 3 of life, generally no therapy is indicated.

Phototherapy (exposure of infant to blue or cool white light) causes photoisomerization of bilirubin to a nontoxic state. Cover infant's eyes.

Indications for use of phototherapy include:
- abnormal rise in the bilirubin level
- when the bilirubin rises early and/or threatens to rise above 20 mg/dl
- prophylaxis in premature infants (less than 1000 grams), severely bruised infants, Rh sensitization, ABO incompatibility

Exchange transfusion is reserved for infants with potentially dangerous levels of serum bilirubin or with the expectation that they will develop potentially dangerous levels. It can correct anemia and lowers the serum bilirubin to approximately one-half the preexchange level. In most instances an umbilical venous and arterial catheter are placed and a single (removes 72% of blood volume) or double (removes 87% of infants blood volume) volume exchange is performed by removing blood and infusing fresh blood in small aliquots.

Hypoglycemia

Defined as a serum glucose level below 30 mg/dl but intermediate symptoms may be seen in infants with serum glucose less than 40 mg/dl.

Etiology

Hyperinsulinism

Infant of diabetic mother

Post exchange transfusion

Islet cell hyperplasia or hyperfunction

Beckwith-Weidemann syndrome

Pancreatic insulin producing tumors

Maternal drug therapy (terbutaline, albuterol, ritodrine, chlorpropamide)

Decreased Glucose Stores
    Intrauterine growth retardation
    Prematurity
Disorders of Metabolism
    Galactosemia
    Adrenal insufficiency
    Congenital hypopituitarism
    Shock
    Asphyxia
    Hypothermia
Sepsis
Polycythemia

Symptoms
Poor feeding
Lethargy
Poor tone
Tremors or seizures
Apnea
Cyanosis
Weak cry

Laboratory Findings
Infants who have an exam consistent with or who are at risk for hypoglycemia should have frequently early measurements of blood glucose. If hypoglycemia is prolonged, or the etiology is unclear, measurements of insulin, growth hormone, cortisol, ACTH and glucagon may be required.

Differential Diagnosis
Heart disease
Maternal - infant drug exposure
Adrenal insufficiency
Hypocalcemic
Hyper or hyponatremia
Renal failure
Liver failure
Sepsis
Asphyxia

Potential Complications
Death
Neurologic injury

Therapeutic Plan

In many instances, early detection and treatment of low serum glucose without true hypoglycemia may avert potential complications.

Infants at risk should have early, frequent feedings with glucose and water until their blood sugar stabilizes.

Glucose 0.5-1.0 gram per kg (given as 25% dextrose in water) may be given by rapid IV infusion. This may be followed by continuous infusion of 4-8 mg of glucose/kg/minute.

Necrotizing Enterocolitis

Significant morbidity and mortality result from this disease, which is primarily associated with premature infants (approximately 5% attack rate). Severity of the disease is related to the degree of necrosis of the bowel wall. Although the disease usually occurs in the first two weeks of life, it can occur as late as two months of age.

Alternate Terminology

NEC

Etiology

Uncertain, but varying factors such as early feeding, polycythemia and hypoperfusion may predispose. An infectious etiology is suggested by the fact that cases sometimes occur in clusters.

Predisposing Conditions

Prematurity, polycythemia, introduction of breast milk or formula, shock or hypoperfusion of the intestines related to a variety of factors such as sepsis and hemorrhage, and perinatal asphyxia.

Pathophysiology

The distal ileum and proximal colon are most frequently involved, with varying degrees of mucosal and/or transmural necrosis. Gas accumulates in the submucosa and may progress to frank necrosis with intestinal wall perforation.

Symptoms

Abdominal distention, emesis or retained feedings, guaiac positive or frankly bloody stools, apnea, shock.

Physical Examination

Varies with severity of illness. The infant initially presents with abdominal distention. Bowel sounds may be absent and evacuation of the stomach may show retained feedings. The infant may be apneic and show signs of poor peripheral perfusion progressing to frank shock with intestinal perforation.

Laboratory Findings

Metabolic acidosis, hypoxemia and hypercapnia may be noted. White count may be elevated or low, anemia and thrombocytopenia may be present.

Differential Diagnosis

Sepsis

Intestinal obstruction

Volvulus

Potential Complications

Peritonitis

Bowel perforation

Sepsis

Shock

Death (5%)

Intestinal stricture (10%)

Short gut syndrome

Diagnostic Plan

Serial roentgenograms of the abdomen should be obtained. Subtle early signs include bowel wall thickening and dilated bowel loops. Pneumatosis intestinalis is diagnostic. If air is noted is the portal vein, the prognosis is poor. Free air may be noted with frank perforation. An abdominal ultrasound may also indicate the pressure of portal vein gas.

Therapeutic Plan

Feeds should be stopped and a nasogastric tube inserted. Fluids and hyperalimentation should be instituted early to maintain adequate nutrition and fluid balance. Cultures of blood, stool and CSF should be obtained and antibiotics begun (aminoglycoside, anti-pseudomonal penicillin and clindcamycin). If hypotension or shock develops, fluid resuscitation is required. If seriously ill, the infant will probably require intubation, and blood gases, CBC, and serum electrolytes should be monitored carefully.

Galactosemia

Disease which may manifest itself in the newborn period with multiple or nonspecific symptoms. Incidence 1:60,000 live births.

Etiology

Deficiency of the enzyme galactose -1- phosphate uridyl transferase which leads to increased concentration of galactose in the blood and urine. There are nine possible mutations which vary in severity.

Pathophysiology

Deficiency of the enzyme inhibits metabolism of galactose - 1- phosphate. Breast milk and standard formula preparations may contain significant amounts of lactose which consists of glucose and galactose. Accumulation of galactose -1- phosphate promotes injury in the liver, brain and kidney.

Symptoms

Vomiting

Hypoglycemia

Lethargy

Feeding problems

Poor weight gain

Convulsions

Physical Examination

Hepatomegaly

Splenomegaly

Jaundice

Cataracts

Ascites

Laboratory Findings

Positive urine reducing substance

Deficient galactose -1 - phosphate uridyl transferase activity in erythrocyte hemolysates

Potential Complications

E coli sepsis

Without early diagnosis, cirrhosis of the liver, cataracts and mental retardation may result.

Therapeutic Plan

Substitution of non-lactose based infant formula at an early age will avoid most complications of this disorder.

Because the infant's mother is heterozygous for this condition, some prenatal injury may occur from transplacental passage of galactose.

Hemorrhagic Disease of the Newborn

Postnatal vitamin K deficiency which may cause life-threatening hemorrhage.

Etiology

Transient decrease in clotting factors II, VII, IX and X occurs in all infant 2 to 3 days after birth, with return to normal levels by 10 days of age.

Pathophysiology

Newborn infants lack intestinal bacterial flora which synthesize vitamin K and have deficient transplacental passage of maternal vitamin K. The bleeding which may occur is primarily confined to the gastrointestinal tract, nares, central nervous system or scalp. Infant boys with vitamin K deficiency may have significant post-circumcision bleeding.

Predisposing Conditions

Prematurity

Maternal use of phenobarbital or phenytoin which may interfere with vitamin K function.

Breast feeding (poor source of vitamin K)

Home births (lack of vitamin K prophylaxis)

Laboratory Findings

Prothrombin, partial thromboplastin and blood coagulations are prolonged. Prothrombin and factors II, VII, IX, and X are decreased.

Differential Diagnosis

Factor XIII and IX deficiency

Disseminated intravascular coagulation

Ingestinal maternal blood

Potential Complications

Intracerebral hemorrhage

Hypovolemia/shock

Death

Therapeutic Plan

Administration of 1 mg of vitamin K intramuscularly at birth prevents the natural decrease of vitamin K-dependent factors in the full term infant. Premature infants and infants born to mothers on phenobarbital or phenytoin, if symptomatic, may require continuous IV infusion of vitamin K and/or transfusion of fresh frozen plasma or whole blood.

Hepatitis in the Neonate

This is a multifactorial disorder which presents as hepatic inflammation.

Etiology

Sepsis, hepatitis B virus, cytomegalovirus, herpes simplex virus, toxoplasmosis, congenital syphilis, and HIV are some of the more common causes. Hepatitis A and C virus are rarely acquired transplacentally or perinatally.

Predisposing Conditions

Maternal infection with any of the above.

Risk factors for sepsis have been outlined previously.

Symptoms
> Vomiting
> Poor feeding
> May also see accompanying signs of disseminated infection with herpes simplex, toxoplasmosis, congenital syphilis, HIV.

Physical Examination
> Jaundice
> Increased hepatic size
> Alteration of consciousness

Laboratory Findings
> Elevated hepatic enzyme levels
> Elevated serum bilirubin
> In instances of significant hepatic dysfunction, coagulation proteins may be decreased and serum ammonia levels may be increased.

Differential Diagnosis
> Biliary atresia
> Cystic fibrosis
> Galactosemia
> Tyrosinosis
> α_1 - antitrypsin deficiency
> Choledochal cyst
> Drug exposure
> Disorders of bile acid metabolism

Potential Complications
> Cirrhosis
> Hepatocellularcarcinoma
> Development of carrier state
> Shock
> Death

Treatment
> Routine prenatal care for expectant mothers can help prevent some causes - mothers should be tested for HBsAg during pregnancy.
>
> Infants born to seropositive mothers should receive hepatitis immune globulin and Hepatitis B vaccine during the first 12 hours after birth with subsequent immunizations at 1 and 6 months.
>
> If a bacterial cause is suspected or identified, appropriate antibiotic coverage should be instituted.

Acyclovir may be used to help treat herpes and varicella viruses.

Famciclovir and foscarnet sodium can be used to treat cytomegalovirus.

Mothers who test positive for HIV can be treated with AZT to help prevent intrauterine transmission and should not breast feed their infants.

Peggy J Hines

Adolescents are not a homogenous group.

"Adolescence" is a period of life beginning with puberty and terminating with cessation of somatic growth. It is also a biopsychosocial process that may begin before puberty and extend well beyond the end of somatic growth, in which case it is culturally defined.

Developmental Considerations: Physical, Cognitive and Medical -Legal

Physical Development
 Puberty is the period during which secondary sex characteristics begin to develop.
  Hypothalamic-pituitary Changes
   Nocturnal sleep-related augmentation of pulsatile LH secretion secondary to an increase in pulsatile GnRH release

   Decrease in hypothalamic and pituitary sensitivity to estradiol and testosterone

   Increase in LH and FSH

   In females, the development of a positive ovulation feedback system:
    estrogen $\rightarrow$ increase GnRH $\rightarrow$ LH $\rightarrow$ ovulation
  Adrenal Gland Changes
   Increased secretion of sex hormones; however, these are not necessary for development of secondary sex characteristics.
  Other Pubertal Changes
   Increased insulin secretion
   Increased plasma somatomedin-C
   Increased GHRH

```
┌─────────────────────────────────────────────────────────────────┐
│                 Pubertal Development Highlights                   │
│                                                                   │
│  Female                          Male                             │
│                                                                   │
│  Starts at age 8-13 years        Starts at age 9.5 - 13.5 years   │
│                                                                   │
│  Duration:  3-4 years            Duration:  about 3 years         │
│                                                                   │
│  Breast development typically    Testicular enlargement is the    │
│    precedes pubic hair             first change                   │
│    development                                                    │
│                                                                   │
│  Adult height reached in:        Adult height reached in latter   │
│    mid-puberty                     half of puberty                │
│                                                                   │
└─────────────────────────────────────────────────────────────────┘
```

Sexual Maturation Stages (Tanner Staging)

Female Breast Development

Stage	I	No glandular tissue, areola conforms to the chest line
Stage	II	Breast bud forms, areola widens and elevates
Stage	III	Continued enlargement of breast bud; further elevation and enlargement of the areola; no separation of breast contours
Stage	IV	Areola and papilla form a mound projecting from the breast contour
Stage	V	Breast adult size (variable); areola and breast in same plane with papilla (nipple) projecting above areola

Pubic Hair Development (male and female)

Stage	I	No pubic hair.
Stage	II	Small amount of long, slightly pigmented hair along base of scrotum and penis in the male or the labia majora in females.
Stage	III	Moderate amount of more curly, pigmented and coarser hair. Begins to spread laterally and over mons pubis.
Stage	IV	Resembles adult hair in coarseness and curliness. Does not extend over medial surface of thighs.
Stage	V	Adult type and quantity extending to medial thigh and in 80% of males along the linea alba .

Male Genitalia Development

Stage	I	Prepubertal, testes less than 1.5 cc in volume.
Stage	II	Testes enlarge, scrotal skin is thinner and reddish and scrotum is larger.
Stage	III	Testes and scrotum continue to grow. Length of penis increases.
Stage	IV	Testes and scrotum continue to grow, scrotum darkens, penis grows in width and length. The glans develops.
Stage	V	Testes, scrotum and penis are adult in size and shape.

Other Physical Pubertal Changes

Height Growth   Pubertal growth accounts for 20-25% of final adult height
Growth spurt is highly variable
Average growth spurt lasts 24-36 months

Weight Growth   Pubertal weight gain accounts for 50% of an individual's ideal adult body weight

Male/Female Differences
Peak height velocity occurs about 18-24 months earlier in the female.
Peak height velocity in females averages 2 cm/year less than in the male.
Peak weight and height velocities coincide in males.

Psychosocial Development in Adolescents

Tasks of Adolescence
•   Achieving independence from parents.
•   Adopting peer codes and lifestyles.
•   Assigning increased importance to body image and accepting one's body image.
•   Establishing sexual, ego, vocational and moral identities.

Task	Early Adolescence	Mid-Adolescence	Late Adolescence
Independence	Less interest in parental activities	Conflict with parents peaks	Reacceptance of parents values
Body Image	Preoccupation with self and pubertal changes	General acceptance of body	Acceptance of pubertal changes
Peers	Intense relationships with same-sex friends	Peak peer group involvement	Peer group less important
	Conformity to peer group values	More time spent in sharing intimate relationships	Increased sexual activity and experimentation
Identity	Increased ability to reason abstractly	Increased scope of feelings	Rational and realistic conscience
	Increased need for privacy	Increased scope of feelings	Sense of perspective
	Idealistic	Increased creative and intellectual activities	Ability to delay, set limits
	Test authority	Feelings of omnipotence and immortality	Practical vocational goals
			Refinement of moral, religious and sexual values

Legal Issues of Adolescence in the United States

A **Mature minor** is an individual who appears to understand risks and benefits of services provided, and who, in the opinion of the health care provider, is of sufficient intellect and maturity to have that understanding.

39

Emancipated minors are individuals aged 16 years and older who are married, joined the armed services, or are living on their own and are managing their own financial affairs.

State Laws vary in rights of adolescents to receive care without parental consent. Most allow mature minors to obtain treatment for drug abuse, physical and sexual abuse, sexually-transmitted diseases and pregnancy-related issues without parental consent.

Confidentiality is a central part of adolescent care. It may be breached when life is at risk.

Diagnostic Modalities

History
Open-ended approach, questionnaires, look for hidden agenda HEADSS interview (Home, Education, Activities, Drugs, Sex, Suicide)

Physical
Height, weight, blood pressure, vision and hearing testing
Skin: acne, facial hair
Eyes: myopia
Dentition: Dental caries, third set of molars
Neck: Thyroid, adenopathy
Breast: Development, masses, gynecomastia
Heart Sounds: Murmurs, clicks
Musculoskeletal: Scoliosis
Genitalia:
- Male

  Stage of development, urethral discharge, scrotal or testicular masses. Inguinal hernia or adenopathy.
- Female

  Stage of development, Pelvic exam yearly for all sexually active adolescents and as indicated.

Laboratory Tests
Hgb/Hct: look for anemia in adolescent females secondary to menses and poor diet.

Urine Analysis: check for asymptomatic proteinuria, hematuria, glucosuria
Rubella Titer: in females prior to becoming pregnant
PPD
Cholesterol: draw level in all at-risk individuals based on family history

In Sexually Active Teenagers
- Females
    * annual Pap smear
      cervical gonorrhea culture
    * Chlamydia screening
    * syphilis serology
    * vaginal wet mount
    * pregnancy testing as indicated
- Heterosexual Males
    * annual syphilis serology
    * urethral cultures for gonorrhea
    * Chlamydia screening
- Homosexual Males
    * annual syphilis serology
    * urethral, rectal and pharyngeal gonorrhea cultures
    * hepatitis B screening
    * HIV testing
    * Chlamydia screening

Disease Profiles

Menstrual Disorders
Amenorrhea
Primary Amenorrhea: no episodes of spontaneous uterine bleeding by 14-16 years of age with absent secondary sexual characteristics; or by 16-18 years of age regardless of normal secondary sexual characteristics.
Secondary Amenorrhea: after previous uterine bleeding, no subsequent menses for 6 months or length of time equal to 3 previous cycles.

CHAPTER 3

Evaluation of Amenorrhea

    Primary Amenorrhea

Evaluation is directed toward determination of pubertal maturation and the presence or absence of internal genitalia. A bimanual pelvic or ultrasound, if necessary, should be done to establish the presence or absence of a uterus and ovaries. The results can then be used to focus on a cause of the amenorrhea as depicted in the following:

	UTERUS ABSENT	UTERUS PRESENT

BREASTS ABSENT	Conclusion: genetic males; gonads produce Muellerian-inhibiting factor but do not produce enough testosterone to induce normal male internal and external genitalia
	
	Karyotype (XY)
	  Gonadal enzyme deficiency
	  Agonadism (testicular regression)
		Conclusion: lack of ovarian estrogen production. Muellerian system developed normally
		
		Follicle Stimulating Hormone low:
		  Hypogonadotropic hypogonadism
		    Lesions of the CNS
		    Kallman syndrome
		    Pituitary gonadotropic deficiencies
		      (chronic disease, anorexia
		      nervosa)
		Follicle Stimulating Hormone high:
		  Gonadal dysgenesis
		    45, XO (Turner syndrome)
		    Other X chromosome variants
		    Pure XX or XY dysgenesis
		    Gonadal enzyme deficiency

BREASTS PRESENT	Conclusion: Genetic male with androgen insensitivity or genetic female with uterine agenesis.
	
	Karyotype:
	
	Female (XX)
	  Muellerian agenesis or hypoplasia
	  Mayer-Rokitansky-Kuster-Hauser syndrome
	
	Male (XY)
	  Androgen insensitivity (testicular
	    feminization)
		Conclusion: Normal phenotypic female with normal Muellerian and pubertal development. Absent menses is due to outlet obstruction or lack of endometrial development and shedding.
		
		Cyclic pain present:
		  Rule out vaginal obstruction
		    imperforate hymen
		    transverse vaginal septum
		
		Cyclic pain absent:
		  Hypothalamic-pituitary-ovarian axis
		    disturbance (evaluate as secondary
		    amenorrhea)

Secondary Amenorrhea

Always consider pregnancy as a cause even if the history given does not suggest the diagnosis. Once pregnancy has been ruled out, the evaluation focuses on the hypothalamic-pituitary-ovarian axis.

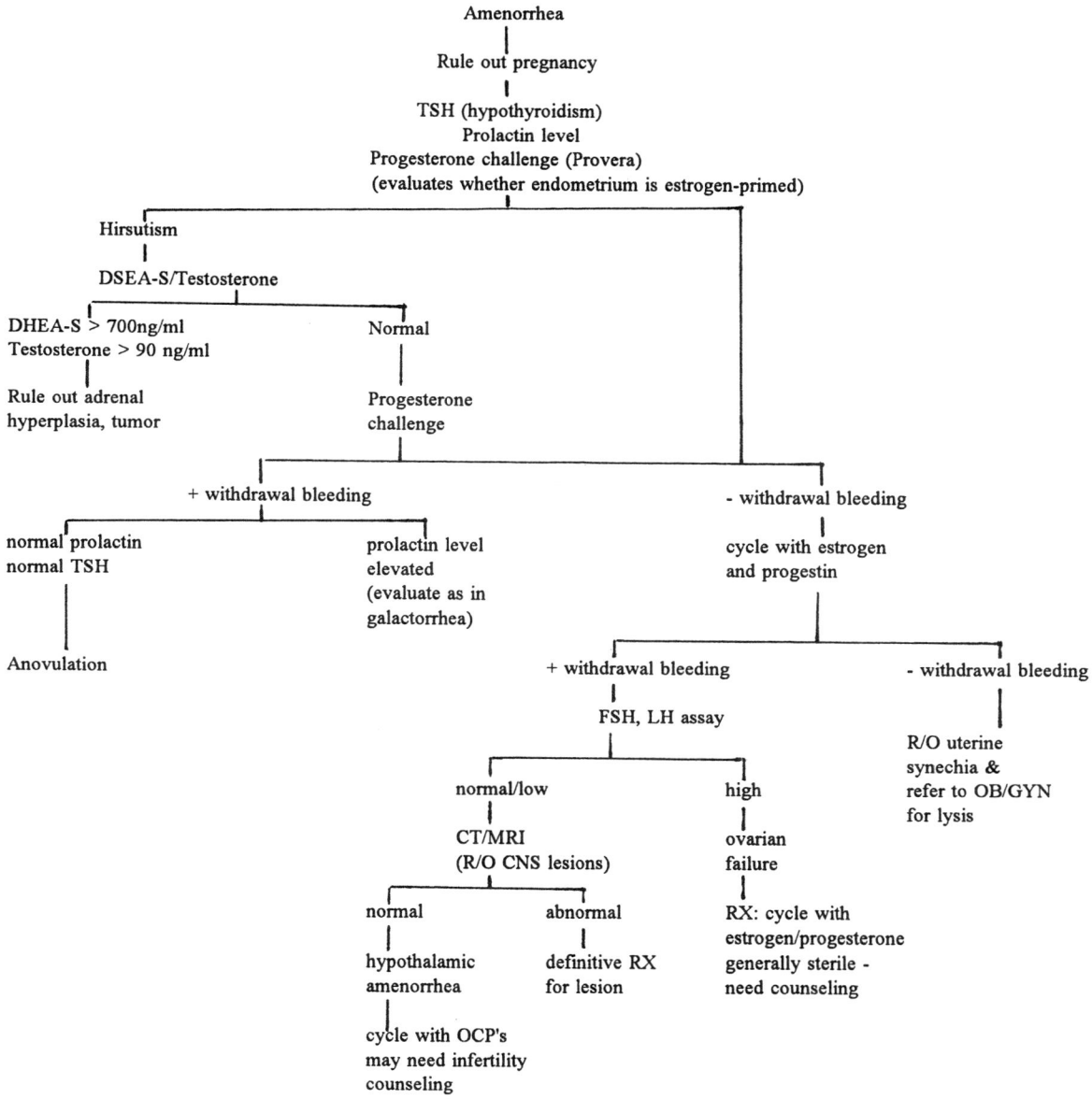

Dysmenorrhea

Painful menstruation
Most common gynecologic problem in adolescence; occurs in 75% of menstruating women.

Etiology
Primary Dysmenorrhea: No identifiable pelvic pathology
Symptoms can be explained by the action of uterine prostaglandins (PGF2 alpha, PGE2 alpha, and cyclic endoperoxidases)

Secondary dysmenorrhea: pain from endometriosis, infection or uterine fibroids

Evaluation
History
timing, character, and location of pain
past history of pelvic infection, intermenstrual bleeding, last menstrual period

Pelvic Exam
abnormal uterine position or shape suggests a uterine malformation (fibroids rare in adolescents)
cervical cultures (chronic pelvic inflammatory disease may present as dysmenorrhea)

Differential Diagnosis
Endometriosis
PID
Benign uterine tumors
Anatomic abnormalities of the uterus

Treatment of Primary Dysmenorrhea
Oral Contraceptives (reduce growth of endometrium and therefore decrease uterine prostaglandin production)
Prostaglandin Inhibitors (block production of prostaglandins)
Mefenamic acid, naproxen, ibuprofen

Dysfunctional Uterine Bleeding
Abnormal endometrial bleeding in the absence of structural pelvic pathology, usually associated with anovulation.

Pathophysiology
Estrogen stimulation of endometrium by corpus luteal progesterone causing overgrowth of the endometrium with patchy desquamation and sloughing.

Evaluation

Immediate goals -- assess hemodynamic stability and identify site of bleeding.

History

Bleeding disorder in patient or family?

History of easy bruising, epistaxis, gums bleeding?

Contraceptive use, IUD?

Sexual history, possibility of pregnancy?

Physical Exam

Vital signs (orthostatic evaluation)

Pelvic exam

evidence of trauma

vaginal foreign body

ovarian masses

signs of PID

signs of pregnancy

Laboratory

CBC

Pregnancy test

Wet prep of vaginal discharge

Cervical cultures for gonorrhea, Chlamydia

Thyroid studies, LFTs, clotting studies as indicated

Differential Diagnosis

Complications of pregnancy (ectopic, abortion, placental polyp)

Endometritis

Malignancy

Cervical lesion, cervicitis

Vaginal pathology (infection, polyp, foreign body, trauma)

Ovarian dysfunction (polycystic ovarian syndrome, infection, tumors)

Systemic disease (blood dyscrasias, cirrhosis, endocrine disorders)

Iatrogenic (OCP's, tranquilizers, IUD)

Management (based on severity of bleeding)

Mild: Inconvenient, unpredictable bleeding; hematocrit normal

Consider oral contraceptive

Reassurance

Menstrual calendar

Reevaluate in 3-6 months

Moderate: Irregular, prolonged, heavy bleeding; mild anemia (Hgb > 10g/dl)

Hormonal therapy

Medroxyprogesterone acetate OR oral contraceptives

Iron supplementation

Menstrual calendar

Reevaluate every 1-3 months

Severe: Irregular, prolonged, heavy bleeding; moderate anemia (Hgb < 10g/dl)

Not actively bleeding

Iron supplementation

Oral contraceptive

Reassurance

Reevaluate every 1-3 months

Actively bleeding

Hospitalize

Transfuse if indicated

Hormonal therapy

Conjugated estrogens IV q 4 hours X 6, concurrent norgestrel/ethinynl estradiol 1 tablet q 6 hours to be followed by OCP's for 6-12 months

OR

Norgestrel/ethinyl estradiol 1 tablet q 6 hours for 24-48 hours followed by OCP's for 6-12 months.

Dilatation and curettage if hormonal therapy fails

Reevaluate every month

Breast Disorders

Asymmetry

Initial breast development may be asymmetric.

Asymmetry may be due to congenital absence of breast tissue.

Associated defects: absence of pectoral muscles or rib defects.

Treatment: Surgical treatment after puberty is finished to allow for full development and equalization.

Accessory Breast Tissue

Most common breast anomaly.

Occurs in 1-2% of females.

Usually located on milk line, most commonly below breast on chest or upper abdomen.

Breast Masses

Most masses found in adolescence are benign

Fibroadenoma

Benign neoplasm of mammary gland.

Most common breast lesion in middle and early female adolescents (76 - 90% of benign lesions).

Physical Findings

Firm, smooth, discrete mobile mass, lateral portion of breast commonly.

Usually less that 5 cm in diameter.

Multiple in 10 - 15%

Fibrocystic Disease

Proliferation of stromal and epithelial elements of breast tissue with ductal dilatation and cyst formation following in many individuals.

Pathophysiologic Abnormality

Fibrocystic changes induced by excess estrogen in relation to progesterone. Some studies implicate Methylxanthines.

Symptoms

Tenderness, increased in late menstrual cycle.

Physical Findings

Cysts usually small, bilateral, firm, mobile. Nodularity - hard and tender areas, 1 - 2 mm to 1 cm in size.

Management of Breast Lesions in Adolescents

Reassure adolescent that lesion is most likely benign. If breast mass feels cystic, aspiration can be done. Consider surgical removal of solid masses greater than 2-3 cm in diameter. Observe most masses for at least 2 - 3 months before intervention - resolution may occur following menstrual cycle. Mammography is not helpful in most cases. Never biopsy or excise a possible breast bud.

Gynecomastia

Excessive development of male mammary glands.

Etiology

Unknown, possibly an increase in biologically active estrogen or increased sensitivity to estrogen. Peak prevalence of 64% at age 14 years.

Pathology

Either 1) ductal proliferation and lobular formation or 2) stromal changes with fibrosis.

Symptoms

Tenderness on palpation in some.

Physical Findings

Type I	One or more subareolar nodules, freely mobile
Type II	Breast nodules beneath the areola and extending beyond the areolar perimeter.
TypeIII	Resembles breast development of sexual maturity stage 3 in female.

Also Look For

Findings suggestive of hypogonadism, hyper or hypothyroidism.

Testicular mass or atrophy.

Findings suggestive of liver disease.

Differential Diagnosis

Drug exposure (estrogen, testosterone, phenothiazines, digoxin, tricyclics, phenytoin)

Renal failure

Recovery from malnutrition

Hypergonadotropic hypogonadism -- Klinefelter's syndrome.

Hyper- or hypothyroidism

Tumors (testicular, bronchogenic, pituitary, adrenal, Hodgkins, hepatomas)

Liver disease

Pseudogynecomastia (secondary to adipose in obese males or increased muscle tissue in the athletic).

Diagnostic Plan

In healthy pubertal males with normal growth no tests are indicated. If gynecomastia occurs before the onset or after the completion of puberty, consider:

Karyotype

HCG level -- may be increased in various carcinomas

Serum estradiol -- feminizing adrenal tumors

Prolactin level, skull films -- pituitary tumors

Thyroid or liver function tests

Chest X-ray -- pulmonary tumors

Therapeutic Plan: Rule out other causes as above --
Reassurance and explanation
Consider surgery for massive gynecomastia or if it causes severe psychological problems.

Galactorrhea

Abnormal milky or watery discharge from one or both breasts in a nonpubertal breast.
Microscopic examination of discharge demonstrates fat goblets.

Etiology

Disruption of hypothalamic-pituitary control of prolactin secretion.

Differential Diagnosis

Drug use

* tranquilizers, reserpine, methyldopa, opiates - lead to decreased dopamine secretion. Dopamine inhibits prolactin secretion.
* oral contraceptives - secondary to LH and FSH suppression and increase in baseline prolactin.

Hypothyroidism - elevated TRH increases prolactin secretion.

Pituitary Causes - Adenomas (micro < 10 mm, macro > 10 mm)
Empty sella syndrome
Acromegaly
Hypothalamic Lesions - Tumors
Infection
Idiopathic
Infiltrative disorders (sarcoid, histiocytosis)
Chest wall manipulation (manual, surgery, trauma, infection)

Endocrine - Cushings disease, Acromegaly

Chronic Renal Disease - decreased clearance of prolactin.

Tumor with ectopic secretion of prolactin.

Diagnostic Plan

Eliminate drugs associated with elevated prolactin.
Serum prolactin level (levels > 100 associated with pituitary adenomas).
TSH level -- rule out thyroid disorders
MRI/CT scan of head when prolactin levels elevated.

Treatment: Based on Etiology
Discontinue drug use if this is the cause.
Treat underlying hypothyroidism.
Microadenoma: bromocriptine --
    Follow prolactin levels q 6 months
    Repeat MRI/CT scan in 6 months, then q 2 - 3 years
Macroadenoma: Surgical removal if mass effect is present or bromocriptine
    ineffective --
    Follow prolactin levels q 6 months.
    Repeat MRI/CT scan q 6 months.

Scrotal Disorders

Scrotal Swelling and Masses
   History
Pain - abrupt onset suggests torsion.
Trauma
Change in testicular size.
Sexual activity: epididymitis is rare without sexual activity.
Prior history of pain: torsion may be preceded by episodes of mild pain.
   Examination
Inspection
•   Testis higher than other suggests torsion, infected testis often lower.
Palpation
•   If pain alleviated by scrotal elevation, consider epididymitis or
    orchitis. No change in pain, suspect torsion.
Painless Masses
•   Assess location: tumor associated with testes.
•   Varicocele : "bag of worms"; more common on left spermatic cord
•   Spermatocele or hydrocele: mass near epididymis
•   Transilluminate:
        clear - hydrocele, spermatocele
        absence -- suggests tumor
   Laboratory
UA: Pyuria > 20 WBC/hpf (epididymitis)
Gram stain: Gram-negative diplococci suggests epididymitis. Negative
    Gram stain suggests Chlamydia epididymitis, orchitis or torsion.

Doppler and scans: Doppler flow study crucial in suspected torsion. If not available, surgical exploration is indicated. Flow will be decreased to torsed testicle.

Differential Diagnosis

Painless scrotal mass or swelling:

Hydrocele

Spermatocele

Varicocele -- prevalence 5 - 15% in 10 - 20 year age group.

Hernia

Testicular tumor -- 2.3/100,000 males, risk increased with history of cryptorchidism.

Idiopathic scrotal edema

Painful scrotal mass or swelling:

Torsion of spermatic cord

Epididymitis

Orchitis

Trauma -- hematoma

Hernia

Torsion of testicular appendage

Management

Torsion: Immediate surgery within 6 hours of symptom onset.

Epididymitis: Scrotal support

Bedrest

Ceftriaxone and Doxycycline (cover for gonorrhea and Chlamydia)

Refer to urologist if symptoms do not resolve.

Testicular tumors (most common solid tumor in males 15 - 35 years old):

Biopsy for confirmative diagnosis and cell type.

Definitive therapy based on biopsy.

Hydrocele: No therapy unless --

• tense hydrocele reduces circulation to the testes.

• bulky mass is uncomfortable or uncosmetic.

Definitive therapy is resection of the parietal tunica vaginalis.

Varicocele: No therapy unless --

• condition is painful.

• massive distention exists.

• involved testis is significantly smaller than the other.

Spermatocele: No therapy indicated.

Sexually Transmitted Diseases

Disease/ Organism	Clinical Presentation	Diagnosis	Treatment	Complication/ Sequelae
Nongonococcal Urethritis • *Chlamydia trachomatis* 40% • *Ureaplasma urealyticum* 30% • *Mycoplasma genitalium* 10% • *Trichomonas vaginalis*	Males: Dysuria Frequency Mucoid to purulent urethral discharge. Some asymptomatic.	WBCs on Gram stain of discharge. + Chlamydia FA/culture - gonorrhea culture	Doxycycline, Tetracycline, or Erythromycin for 7 days or Azithromycin Refer/℞ partner Use condoms	Urethral strictures Prostatitis Epididymitis
Mucopurulent Cervicitis • *Chlamydia trachomatis* • *Neisseria gonorrheae* • *Herpes simplex virus*	Females: Asymptomatic or yellow mucopurulent endocervical exudate	Exudate on endocervical swab > 20 PMNs/HPF on Gram stain of endocervical discharge. + Chlamydia culture/FA + GC culture	Ceftriaxone IM or Cefixime PO PLUS Doxycycline or Erythromycin Consider Amoxicillin if pregnant Refer/℞ partner Use condoms	Salpingitis PID Conjunctivitis, pneumonia in newborn.
Condyloma acuminata (genital warts) Human papillomavirus	Single or multiple soft, fleshy growths on perineum, perianally on cervix, intravaginally.	Visual colposcopy Pap smear	Cryotherapy Podophyllin (not in pregnancy) TCA Electrocautery Examine sexual partner	Obstruction of vagina Infection of newborn (uncommon) Cervical cancer

Gonorrhea	Males: Dysuria, purulent urethral discharge. Females: Vaginal discharge, abnormal menses, lower abdominal pain. Look for pharyngeal and rectal infection.	Microscopic identification of Gm-negative diplococci on urethral exudate or endocervical material. Positive culture.	Ceftriaxone IM or Cefixime and Doxycycline or Erythromycin Spectinomycin IM for penicillin allergic patients Refer/℞ partner Use condoms	PID Epididymitis Sterility
PID (Pelvic inflammatory disease)	Females: Pain, tenderness in lower abdomen, cervix, uterus, adnexa. Fever, chills, increased sed rate, WBC. Hx: multiple sexual partners, past history of PID, IUD. R/O ectopic pregnancy, appendicitis	Definitive visualization of inflamed fallopian tubes and positive culture of tubal exudate at laparoscopy. Presumptive - clinical presentation +/- positive cultures.	Outpatient: Cefoxitin/ Probenecid or Ceftriaxone PLUS Doxycycline or Erythromycin for 14 days Inpatient: Doxycycline BID PLUS Cefoxitin IV q 6 OR Clindamycin PLUS Gentamicin. Refer/℞ partner	Ectopic pregnancy Abscess Involuntary infertility Recurrent PID Recurrent Pelvic Pain
Pediculosis *Phthirus pubis* (pubic louse)	Itching, erythematous papules, nits or adult lice on pubic hairs	Exam - lice or nits on pubic hair	Lindane, clean linen in hot water. Treat partner.	Excoriation lymphadenitis pyoderma

Herpes Genitalis (*Herpes Simplex* Virus, Types I and II)	Single or multiple vesicles of genitalia. Rupture leads to painful ulcers	Presumptive history, typical lesions, multinucleated giant cells on Pap smear Definition: HSV tissue culture showing cytopathic effects	No known cure Palliative: Acyclovir with 1st episode Annual Pap smears Evaluate partner	Fetal Wastage infection of newborn. Urethral stricture
Syphilis *Treponema pallidum*	Primary - classical chancre is painless, indurated. Suspect syphilis in all genital lesions Secondary - skin rash (palms and soles) *Condyloma lata,* Lymphadeno-pathy Latent - 0 clinical signs	Presumptive - Primary: typical lesion and newly positive serologic test, or titer of serologic test for syphilis 4 fold greater that last titer. Secondary: presentation and strongly reactive serological test. Definitive: + dark field examination of material from lesion or lymph node.	Primary, Secondary, early syphilis < 1 year: Benzathine Penicillin or if allergic to Penicillin use Doxycycline or Erythromycin Evaluate and Ŗ partner	Congenital Syphilis Cardiovascular Syphilis Neurologic involvement
Chancroid *Hemophilus ducreyi*	Single, superficial painful ulcer, inguinal bubo (25 - 60%)	Presumptive - clinical presentation (R/O syphilis) Definitive - culture + for *H. ducreyi*	Erythromycin or Ceftriaxone Evaluate/Ŗ partner	Secondary infection of ulcer Buboes may rupture causing fistula.

Molluscum Contagiosum (DNA virus from Poxvirus group)	1-5mm smooth, rounded, shiny, firm papules, with umbilicated centers	Presentation -- microscopic exam of material from lesion reveals molluscum inclusive bodies	Curettage Cryotherapy Evaluate/℞ partner	Secondary infection

Reproductive Issues

Half of all adolescents are sexually active by 17 years of age. < 1/3 use any effective form of birth control. A significant percent of some subgroups are sexually active by age 12-14 years (homeless, juvenile court, etc.)

Contraception

Oral Contraceptive Pill - Most common form used by adolescents.
Failure rate 2 - 4%.

Mechanism of Action - Suppresses ovulation, decreases likelihood of implantation, makes cervical mucus hostile to sperm.

Contraindications to use in adolescents -

Absolute -- Hypertension
History of thromboembolic disease, cerebrovascular accident.
Undiagnosed abnormal genital bleeding.
Relative - Borderline hypertension
Migraine headaches
Diabetes
Sickle Cell Disease
(Keep in perspective: eg, what are the risks for a 16-year-old pregnant diabetic vs. risk of OCPs.)
Common side effects -
Breakthrough bleeding.
Nausea
Weight gain
Headaches
Mood swings

Advantages - decreased menstrual flow
Decreased dysmenorrhea
Improvement of acne
Evaluation prior to starting Pill -
Screen for risk factors
Complete physical examination
Pelvic examination
Weight and blood pressure check
Laboratory Pap smear, gonorrhea culture, Chlamydia FA or culture, RPR and pregnancy test if indicated.
Barrier Methods - used by < 20% of adolescents.
Failure rate 10 - 20%.

Mechanism of action - Prevent sperm from entering uterus

No contraindications to use.

Types
Diaphragm
Cervical Cap
Condom

IUD - not usually recommended in sexually active teenagers.

Injectable Progesterone - most commonly used contraception outside the United States.
Given every 3 months IM
Side effects: amenorrhea/dysfunctional uterine bleeding/weight gain
Norplant - available; 5 year duration of action; stringent guidelines should be followed to determine best candidates.

Mechanism of action - suppresses ovulation

Indications for use - significant contraindication to estrogen use exists.
- Patient unwilling to use barriers contraceptives or the pill.
- When all other forms of contraception have failed and pregnancy is not desired.
- Adolescent is mentally unable to understand the meaning of pregnancy and is unable to use other forms of contraception.

Acne

Major skin problem in adolescents

Pathophysiology

Androgens produced during puberty cause increased sebum production from the sebaceous gland. Bacteria in the follicles attract a white leukocyte response. WBC activity then releases hydrolytic enzymes which cause a local inflammatory reaction. Resolution may leave scarring.

Definition of Lesions

Comedo - hyperkeratosis of follicular epithelium.

- Whiteheads - closed comedones resulting in elevated papules in the skin.
- Blackheads - later stage of enlarged comedones that contain melanin; when they eventually open, it leads to inflammatory changes.
- Cystic acne - not cysts; they are composed of nodules resulting in erythematous papules (pimples) or pus-filled papules (pustules).

Treatment

Goal is to decrease sebum production and decrease bacterial activity.

- Comedolytic and Antikeratolytic Agents
    * topical retinoic acid
    * benzoyl peroxide
- Antibacterial Agents
    * topical and systemic antibiotics (tetracycline, erythromycin)
- Sebaceous Gland Inhibitor
    * systemic isotretinoin
    * oral contraceptives
- Surgical removal of comedones and scars
- Exfoliating Agents
    * ultraviolet light
    * cryotherapy

Mental Health Issues

Depression

60% of teenagers surveyed said they experienced depression once a month to daily. More common in women than men.

Etiology
- Change in peer and/or dating relationships
- Family influences, problems with parents
- Poor school experiences: bad grades, conflict with teachers, peer conflict
- Poor self image

Clinical Features
- Recurrent somatic complaints
- Mood swings
- Decline in school performance
- Apathy

Therapy
- Counseling for family and teenager
- May consider antidepressant, but be cautious

Suicide
- 3rd most common cause of death in adolescents
- Suicide attempts outnumber successful suicides 50-200/1
- Females make more attempts
- Males more often succeed
- 60% of teenagers who commit suicide have made a previous attempt

Preventive Steps
- All adolescents should be asked about suicidal thought.
- If suicidal thoughts are present, assess risk
  - * review history of suicide/suicide attempts
  - * assess level of family support and recognition of problem
  - * teenager recovering from depression is more likely to commit suicide
  - * danger signs
    - ▷ getting affairs in order giving things away
    - ▷ withdrawal from family/friends
    - ▷ history of suicide or alcohol abuse in family
    - ▷ precipitating events:
      - ◇ break-up with significant other
      - ◇ conflict with peers
      - ◇ pregnancy
      - ◇ conflict with parents (most common)

Therapy
- Team approach - physician, social worker, psychiatrist or psychologist
- Ambulatory Treatment
  * no significant past history
  * method used less lethal
  * suicide attempt occurred when help was available
  * family is supportive and recognizes problem
  * mental health care worker is available
  * patient and family willing to follow-up
- Hospitalization Necessary
  * safe environment needed
  * family not supportive
  * past history of suicide attempt
  * history of depression
  * method used was lethal or medical care needed
  * attempt occurred without warning
  * ambulatory services not available

Substance Abuse

Stages
Stage I - Experimentation
Starts with peers, under peer pressure.
Few behavioral changes.
User experiences euphoria and guilt.
Stage II - Abuse to Relieve Stress
More than occasional use.
Occurs in nonsocial settings.
Supply of substance maintained.
Peer group develops around substance abuse.
Stage III - Regular Abuse
User involved in drug-oriented culture.
Most peers use drugs. Problem behavior chronic.
May have trouble with the law.
User depressed when not using drugs.
User needs to raise money to support habit.

Stage IV - Dependence

Drug used to prevent depression, not to produce euphoria.

Adolescent may drop out of school.

Physical changes such as weight loss, fatigue, blackouts and chronic cough may occur.

Therapy

Stages I and II may be treated on an outpatient basis.

Stages III and IV require hospitalization and/or placement in residential rehabilitation facility.

Elias Srouji
Kendall Stanford
Roger Thompson

Chronically Recurring Problems In Ambulatory Pediatrics

Multiple perplexing problems will tend to surface over and over again in the pediatric clinic setting. Many of these visits are simply due to the parent's or child's need to know if they need to worry and/or just how much they should worry.

The clinician's role is to sort through the parent's and patient's frustrations and fears to find out what are their real concerns. Attempts should then be made to systematically evaluate whether there is a need for concern. If so, where do we go from here? If not, give parents permission to quit worrying or at least decrease their fears. But do not be trapped into diagnosis by becoming fixated on the parent's or patient's perception of the problem.

Remember that all problems do not need to be solved in a single visit. Most of these problems have more than one method of treatment. Some of these problems may never be totally cured.

The following are several of the common perplexing problems that are seen frequently in ambulatory pediatrics.

Diurnal Enuresis (Daytime Wetting)
Definition
Lack of bladder control during waking hours in a child old enough to maintain bladder control.
- **Primary Enuresis** - untrained after 2 1/2 years in a developmentally normal child
- **Secondary Enuresis** - previously toilet trained, then regresses
  * usually voids the entire contents of bladder
  * occasional seepage of a few drops probably normal
  * occasional wetting during the first two years post training; not abnormal - usually associated with postponement of voiding secondary to playing, etc.

Etiology
- Organic Causes (5% of children with daytime wetting)
  * #1 cause - urinary tract infections; often associated with frequency and dysuria; females who use bubble bath may develop daytime wetting associated with a distal chemical urethritis
  * ectopic ureter - if patient has continual wetness

* neurogenic bladder; often associated with gait disturbance and poor bowel control
* lower urinary tract obstruction leads to bladder distension and overflow incontinence; history of straining at urine, dribbling, or small caliber stream suggests this condition
* pelvic masses (such as presacral teratoma, hydrocolpos or fecal impaction); pressure on bladder may lead to stress incontinence with running, coughing, or lifting
* Physiologic Causes
  * vaginal reflux - after voiding, urine seeps out of vagina; most common with obese girls
  * giggle incontinence - detrusor instability (> 90% female); bladder spasms leading to abrupt voiding; many have associated nocturnal enuresis
* Psychogenic
  * stress-related; usually between the ages of two and six years; associated with fear or anxiety (eg, birth of a sibling, loss of a relative, school-related problems) - irregular, infrequent
  * resistive child; a child greater than two and one-half years who has not responded to toilet training; resistive and negative about using the toilet; most are boys; often associated with a high-pressure approach to toilet training, including severe physical punishment

Incidence
* approximately 1% in 7 - 12 year olds
* 50 - 60% of these have associated nocturnal enuresis

Evaluation
* History: dysuria, frequency, hematuria, continuous dampness vs intermittent flow, previous UTI, precipitating events, use of punishment or coercion, associated nocturnal enuresis or encopresis
* Physical Exam
  * abdominal exam - rule out bladder distension or fecal impaction
  * genital exam - perianal sensation, anal tone, assessment of pressure and shape of urine stream (Lays)
  * lower back for spinal abnormalities
* Laboratory: urinalysis, urine culture
* If positive physical findings or recurrent UTI, refer for urologic consultation

Management

Treat daytime incontinence before nocturnal

- urgency incontinence - stream interruption exercises
- stress related - sympathy, support; ask for school cooperation in reducing tension
- resistive child - discontinue punishment; offer positive reinforcement for success; encourage positive interaction between parent and child

Nocturnal Enuresis

Definition

The involuntary passage of urine during sleep *occurring greater* than one time per month in a child older than 3 years.

Incidence

- 30%   at age 4
- 10%   at age 6
- 3%   at age 12
- 1%   at age 18

Risk Factors

- familial predisposition
- males > females; 60% vs 40%
- most have small functional bladder capacity
- most without emotional problems
- organic etiology in 1-2% (most common UTI)
- spontaneous cure rate 15% per year

Management

- motivational counseling (ages 3-6)
- child takes active role
- reassurance to parents and child
- positive reinforcement for dry nights
- decrease family friction
- decrease fluids three hours prior to bedtime and encourage voiding just prior to bedtime
- follow-up to give reinforcement
- bladder exercises (ages 6 - 8)
  - * bladder stretching
  - * stream interruption
  - * increase early morning fluid intake

- enuresis alarms (greater than 8 years) to awaken child with first drops (good success rate); set alarm clock to waken child approximately four hours after retiring
- Medications (greater than 8 years; use only if other methods have failed)
  - * Imipramine - tricyclic, not recommended secondary to potentially dangerous side effects
  - * Antispasmodics - Ditropan
  - * Antidiuretics - DDAVP

  REMEMBER: Relapses and treatment failures are common.

Encopresis

Definition

Deposition of formed or semiformed stool in the underwear or other abnormal places occurring after the age of four years.

Prevalence

1 - 3 % of school-aged children; boys much greater frequency than girls (86%)

Development of Encopresis

- intermittent stool retention/constipation
- rectum becomes distended
- sensory feedback becomes impaired
- rectal wall becomes stretched and unable to contract effectively
- stools become harder and larger
- painful defecation leads to further retention
- soft stool and mucus begins to seep around impacted stool
- child may pass large-diameter stools

Etiologic Considerations

- early colonic inertia
- constipation from early life
- parental overreaction may aggravate
- child may balk at bowel training
- incomplete training
- critical life events may thwart attempts to develop continence (eg, illness, birth of sibling; loss of family member, etc.)
- the untrained child may continue to soil then retain when faced with social pressures
- toilet aversion; toilet phobia
- situational toilet avoidance; new environment (school, daycare, etc.); lack of privacy (children avoid defecation; constipation and encopresis follow)
- incomplete defecation; partial evacuation results in constipation;

- encopresis common in children with attention deficit disorders
- psychosocial/stress induced; may be a manifestation of family problems (eg, marital strife, abuse, neglect)

Other Causes of Chronic Constipation

- Hirschsprung's disease (aganglionic megacolon) 1:25,000
- spinal cord lesions
- malnutrition
- dietary indiscretions (eg, lack of fiber or overindulgence on cow's milk
- disorders of voluntary muscle function (amyotonia congenita, cerebral palsy, infectious polyneuritis)
- metabolic - infantile renal acidosis, diabetes insipidus, idiopathic hypercalcemia

Evaluation

- thorough history
- complete physical exam including rectal exam
- abdominal X-ray, and barium enema when indicated
- laboratory tests only if suspicion of underlying metabolic disorder
- rectal biopsy if signs of Hirschsprung's

Management

Goal is to attain regular bowel habits and restoration of neuromuscular bowel function.

- demystify - reassure that many children have this problem and that the child often **cannot** feel a bowel movement coming on.
- catharsis
  * clean out procedure; enemas and laxatives
  * follow-up X-ray to prove successful clean out (if necessary)
- establish regular bowel habits; sit 10 minutes at least two times per day after meals
- mineral oil after clean out
- consider need for stool softeners
- increase dietary fiber
- treatment requires long-term commitment; 20% of cases may have recurrence of symptoms; encourage perseverance
- enlist school cooperation; permit bathroom visits when needed; private bathroom if necessary

Recurrent Abdominal Pain (RAP)
Definition

"The presence of at least three discrete episodes of debilitating (abdominal) pain occurring over at least a three-month period during the year preceding the clinical examination." (Apley 1975)

Incidence

10 - 15 percent of school-aged children

Personality Profile

Two categories:

- Super achievers, verbal, obsessive-compulsive, sensitive, "older than their years"
- Average intelligence, but often immature in speech and behavior when compared to more productive sibling

Family History

Often many relatives will have a history of conditions such as irritable colon, spastic colitis, anxiety attacks and mental illness. Positive family history of migraines is also common.

Diagnosis

Organic considerations to be considered in the differential diagnosis:

- Occult constipation of childhood; colonic distension leads to crampy abdominal pain.
- Lactase deficiency
- Malabsorption (including insufficiency and celiac disease)
- Chronic ingestions (eg, lead)
- Medications - salicylates, steroids, and aminophylline; constipating medications such as Ritalin, narcotic cough medications, anticholinergic medications, Dilantin
- abdominal and inguinal hernias
- peptic ulcer disease
- Crohn's disease and ulcerative colitis
- rheumatic and collagen vascular diseases
- Henoch-Schönlein purpura
- hereditary angioneurotic edema
- parasitic infections (eg, giardiases or ascariasis) (Pinworms do not induce pain)
- late complications of trauma or abuse
- gynecological conditions (endometriosis, PID, hematocolpos, etc.)
- metabolic derangements, hyperlipidemias, diabetes, porphyria, hypothyroidism, hypocalcemia (other stigmata of these conditions should be clinically detectable)
- hematologic disorders, sickle cell, hemolytic anemia, leukemias, lymphoma
- neoplasms
- Idiopathic hypercalcuria

Functional Considerations

Some studies show an increased number of stressful events in families of children with RAP, sometimes a recent traumatic event.

Often associated with school phobia. Stress related to school situations may trigger attacks. Height and weight are unaffected.

Assessment

- History
  - * careful assessment of the pain, associated symptoms, triggering events, etc.
  - * past medical history
  - * personality
  - * school attendance and performance
  - * family history
  - * review of systems
- Physical Exam
  - * meticulous - both diagnostic and therapeutic
  - * include rectal and pelvic
- Laboratory
  - * minimum - CBC, sed rate, UA, PPD, stool for blood, ova, and parasites, liver function tests
  - * abdominal ultrasound, X-ray (if indicated)
  - * further tests as indicated

Management

- discuss family concerns; assure parents and child that no major illness is evident
- alter environment as necessary
- discuss the fact that the emotional state can influence the GI tract
- keep diary of episodes and related events
- medicines, laxatives as needed
- DO NOT feel pressured to make a diagnosis on the first visit
- give follow-up and positive reinforcement
- allow time for parent and child separately
- refer for psychological evaluation in confusing or refractory cases

Recurrent Headaches

Incidence and Prevalence

- Nonspecific, Nonrecurrent Headache:
  - * By 7 years, 40%
  - * By 15 years, 75%
- Frequent recurring Headaches
  - * Non migraine, 15.7% by age 15 years
  - * Migraine, 5.3% by age 15 years

- Male : Female
  - * Under 15 years 5.5 : 4.3
  - * Over 15 years 4.6 : 9

Classification: Useful for Evaluation

- Migraine
  - * Without aura (common)
  - * With aura
    - ▷ classic; usual aura visual
    - ▷ complicated:
      - ◇ transient neurological manifestations
      - ◇ basilar artery migrate (vertigo, syncope)
      - ◇ acute confusional
      - ◇ "Alice in Wonderland" severe
- Non Migraine
  - * Tension: often difficult to differentiate from migraine
    - ▷ with psychopathology
    - ▷ without psychopathology
  - * Traction: a small percentage, but with serious implications
    - ▷ intracranial masses
    - ▷ pseudotumor cerebri
  - * Headaches due to diseases of other head and neck structures. eg, eyes (astigmatism, hyperopia), sinusitis, dental diseases, infections, trauma, or allergy. These are rare causes of recurrent headaches in children.

Evaluation

- History (very important)
  - * Antecedent events (trauma, loss, stress, etc.)
  - * Onset
  - * Length of history of headaches
  - * Course over duration: changes in character, intensity and frequency
  - * Frequency of episodes
  - * Intensity and character of pain episodes
  - * Duration of episodes
  - * Location of pain
  - * Presence of warning symptoms (aura)
  - * Associated symptoms and signs
  - * Time of day of start of episodes
  - * Does it require cessation of activity?
  - * Any aggravating factors (positional, etc.)
  - * Any alleviating factors

- * Family history of headaches
- * Psychosocial history
- Physical Examination
  - * Growth parameters and pattern of height curve
  - * Complete examination including blood pressure, skin for neurofibromatosis, phacomatosis
  - * Full neurological examination
  - * Eye examination: visual acuity, visual fields, fundoscopy
- Laboratory: urine specific priority, other as indicated
- Imaging: If indicated, MRI is the optimal

Traction or Brain Tumor Headaches
- Differentiating Characteristics
  - * Progressive course
  - * Occurs early mornings
  - * Position affects intensity
  - * Vomiting
  - * Ocular and/or neurologic signs must be carefully looked for
- Follow Up
  - * When headache is of less than 6 months history, and no symptoms or signs suggestive of traction headaches, patient to be seen at frequent intervals (monthly at least) and reevaluated with complete neurological and fundoscopic exams. (Dilate pupils if needed.)
  - * Otherwise, appropriate imaging: MRI or CT with contrast to be done.
  - * Imaging to be done in any child less than 4 years old with recurrent or persistent headaches.

Migraine
- Criteria for Diagnosis
  - * Migraine without aura
    - ▷ five attacks
    - ▷ duration of 4 to 72 hours
    - ▷ characteristics (two out of four)
      - ◇ unilateral
      - ◇ pulsating
      - ◇ moderate or severe
      - ◇ aggravated by physical activity
    - ▷ concommitant features (one out of two)
      - ◇ nausea and/or vomiting
      - ◇ photophobia and phonophobia

* Migraine with aura
  ▷ two attacks
  ▷ characteristics (three out of four)
     ◇ aura indicating focal cerebral or brainstem dysfunction
     ◇ aura developing gradually over 4 min. or several in succession
     ◇ aura lasting < 60 minutes
     ◇ headache appearing before, with, or within 60 minutes of the aura

Prognosis
- Better than adults: 10-12% remit per year.
- Migraine starting around or beyond puberty may continue into adulthood.

Management
- Non Medicinal Therapies
  * Food avoidance when (rarely) appropriate, elimination of other triggering Factors
     * Biofeedback, Hypnosis, Relaxation
- Medicinal
  * Treatment of Episode
     ▷ Aspirin or Acetaminophen (most commonly used)
     ▷ Ergotamine: not recommended under 12 years, and even then not more than once a week.
     ▷ Midrin
     ▷ Emergency prescription for status or very severe attack:
        ◇ DHE intravenously (dihydroergotamine)
        ◇ Sumatriptan (very little experience in children)
  * Prophylactic treatment: indicated only if migraine attacks are frequent or compromise child's achievements.
     ▷ Beta-adrenergic blockers, eg, Propranolol. Make SURE the patient is not asthmatic.
     ▷ Cyproheptadine

Infantile Colic
  Definition

Paroxysm of irritability, fussing, or crying lasting a total of three hours a day and occurring on more than three days in any one week in an infant less than three months of age.

Incidence

Approximately 10% of infants age one to three months; usually resolves spontaneously by three to four months

Possible Etiologies

- intrinsic problems - temperamental predisposition, low sensory threshold
- extrinsic problems - overstimulating environment, maternal anxiety
- feeding problems - underfed/overfed, excessive air swallowed, inadequate burping, milk allergy

Diagnosis - Is a Diagnosis of Exclusion

- rule out organic causes for excessive crying
- include detailed history, narrative of the infant's typical day, occurrence and progression of symptoms
  * usual crying time late afternoon and evening
  * short-lived remission following any maneuver: change of position, rocking, feeding, etc.
  * usually proper or excessive weight gain

Physical Exam

- thorough exam to rule out evidence of organic pathology
- laboratory seldom indicated

Management

- counseling of parents
  * reassure that infant is healthy
  * empathize
  * discuss parental anxiety and psychosocial stressors
- observe parental handling of infant and intervene appropriately (eg, decrease overstimulation)
- discuss the option of not always picking up child if crying occurs when child is dry and well fed
- medication - controversial, not recommended (Phenobarbital, Bentyl)
- close follow-up and reassurance

Failure to Thrive (FTT)

Definition

A term used to describe infants or young children whose weights are persistently below the third percentile for age on standardized growth charts.

Epidemiology

3% to 5% of infants under one year of age admitted to the hospital; 70% to 80% of these without organic etiology

Etiology

- Non-Organic (most common) inadequate intake the final determinant
  * underlying psychosocial issues may play a large part (psychologic stress can inhibit growth hormone production)
  * emotional deprivation and/or physical abuse or neglect may be involved
  * environmental disruption
- Organic
  * CNS abnormalities
  * malabsorption
  * cystic fibrosis
  * partial cleft palate
  * congenital heart disease
  * endocrine disorders
  * idiopathic hypercalcemia
  * Turner Syndrome and other chromosomal abnormalities
  * renal disease
  * chronic infection
  * rheumatic disorders
  * malignancies

Diagnosis and Evaluation

- Thorough history
  * family history; growth patterns of siblings, etc.; history of organic disease in close family members
  * detailed history of feeding practices and diet (diet diary)
  * close observation of interactions between parents and child
  * detailed growth chart
    ▷ has growth been steady although below the third percentile?
    ▷ was growth normal and suddenly slowed? If so, at what point?
- Thorough physical exam
  * look for signs or symptoms of organic pathology
  * careful assessment of height, weight, and FOC
  * observe for signs of physical and emotional deprivation (eg, apathy, poor hygiene, intense eye contact, withdrawing behavior)
- Developmental assessment
- Laboratory
  * baseline CBC and UA
  * further tests as indicated by history and physical examination
- Period of observation in hospital

Management
- address medical problems
- if inadequate intake, ensure adequate calories for maintenance and catch up growth
- frequent weight checks
- indications for hospitalization: severe malnutrition or dehydration, failure of outpatient management, evidence of abuse or neglect, extreme parental anxiety

Attention Deficit Disorder (ADD)
Definition

Children with short attention span, high distractibility and an inability to ignore extraneous stimuli when trying to attend to a task. They are often impulsive and have difficulty regulating their actions to conform with social norms. They are often hyperactive and have poor frustration tolerance.

Clinical Manifestation
- as in the definition above
- emotional and behavioral difficulties common
- often socially ostracized
- poor self esteem
- increased incidence of learning disabilities
- often reported to be more active than normal from birth on

Diagnosis
- thorough history including performance and teacher's perception of the child
- thorough physical exam including vision, hearing, and neurologic exams (patient may not display their characteristic behavior in the physician's office)
- children with ADD may show increased numbers of "soft" neurologic signs (eg, mixed hand preference, impaired balance, astereognosis, dysdiadochokinesia, and problems in fine motor coordination)
- laboratory not generally helpful
- behavior rating scales - Conners Parent Rating Scale, Conners Teacher Rating Scale to be sent with parents and teacher for rating over a period of several days duration.
- consider referral for psychometric testing when learning difficulties are present

Management
- counseling; helping parents' understand the child's problems
- behavior modification - parent and child
- encourage a structured environment
- medication - stimulants: Methylphenidate (Ritalin); Dextroamphetamine (Dexedrine); Pemoline (Cylert)

* give a clinical trial to reassess with behavior rating scales
* use only in conjunction with counseling and behavior modification
• consider psychotherapy when signs of severe depression or serious affective disturbances are detected

Recurrent Infections
Definition
Infections occurring with a frequency greater than the norm or caused by an unusual or opportunistic organism.

No person escapes their childhood without occasional illness. When does it become necessary to evaluate a child for the possibility of an immune deficiency?

As with most medical encounters, the History and Physical Exam will play the largest role in determining whether a child's infections falls within normal limits or whether further work-up is desirable. Even with a comprehensive H&P it can at times be difficult to decide; all of the following commonly occur in normal childhood:

Bacterial Infections
Meningitis
Acute Otitis Media (multiple organisms)
Pharyngitis
Sinusitis
Pneumonia (unless recurrent or caused by unusual organisms)
Gastroenteritis
Cellulitis
Impetigo
Urinary Tract Infections

Viral Infections
Upper Respiratory Infections (colds)
Lower Respiratory Infections/Bronchiolitis
Gastroenteritis
Viral Syndromes/exanthems

Fungal Infections
Superficial fungal infections
Thrush

Evaluation

Any of the above can occur in completely immunocompetent children and are not a manifestation of an underlying disorder. Underlying immunodeficiencies can arise from defects in the B cells, the T cells, phagocytic defects, or complement defects. If pursuit of an immunodeficiency diagnosis is warranted, the following is reasonable, in addition to an initial CBC, appropriate X-rays, bone scans, cultures and erythrocyte sedimentation rate:

Quantitative immunoglobulin levels: IgG, IgM, IgA; IgG subclasses

Isohemagglutinin titer to measure IgM function

Delayed hypersensitivity skin tests for *Candida*, tetanus toxoid, tuberculin, or antigen to mumps to measure T cell function

Chemiluminescence, nitroblue tetrazolium (NBT) dye test to measure neutrophil function IgE level

Total hemolytic complement (CH50) to measure complement activity C3, C4 levels to measure major complement pathway components

Management

Specific to the etiology.

Denise C Scott

Genetics

Developmental Considerations

There are many genetic causes of human disease. Genetic abnormalities may produce congenital malformations (Trisomy 13, 18), metabolic disturbances (PKU, galactosemia), specific organ dysfunction (mental retardation, congenital heart disease) or abnormalities of sexual differentiation (Turner syndrome).

Approximately 1% of all newborns will manifest monogenic disease, 0.5% will have a chromosomal abnormality and 1-3% will have a multifactorial disease.

When interpreting a structural defect, the clinician is looking back to an early stage in development or morphogenesis. Morphogenesis is genetically determined and environmentally dependent. Each genetic determinant is present in two doses, one from each parent. Of the 23 pairs of chromosomes in each normal human diploid cell, 22 pairs are autosomal chromosomes and one pair is the sex chromosomes.

There are three general genetic causes of abnormal morphogenesis: mutant genes in a single or double dose, gross chromosomal abnormalities (deletions, translocations, duplications, etc.) and polygenic determinants. Polygenic causes probably account for the majority of malformations and are the consequence of multiple minor gene differences at many loci, no one of which is fully responsible for the defect.

Malformations represent abnormalities or incomplete development in tissue formation.

Deformations are due to altered mechanical forces on normal tissue.

Disruption is the result of breakdown of previously normal tissue.

Genetic characteristics of genes are expressed in offspring through Mendelian inheritance patterns:

Autosomal dominant - A single mutant gene (allele) produces an abnormal characteristic (person is heterozygous for defective gene). The risk of the mutant gene being passed to each offspring is 50%.

Autosomal recessive - A mutant gene (allele) produces an abnormal characteristic only when present in a double dose (two identical alleles; person is homozygous for defect). The risk of the mutant genes being passed to any offspring is 25%, the risk of an offspring being a carrier for the mutant gene and being phenotypically affected is 50%.

X-linked inheritance - The mutant gene(s) is located on the X chromosome (may be X-linked recessive or dominant). Dominant forms may be expressed in both males and females. Affected males will have normal sons but all daughters will be affected.

Recessive forms carry a 50% risk for males to be affected and 50% risk of female offspring being carriers. There is no male-to-male transmission.

Indications for obtaining chromosomal (cytogenetic) studies in children include:
- confirmation of a suspected chromosomal syndrome
- multiple organ system malformation
- significant developmental delay or mental retardation
- short stature in a female or very delayed menarche
- ambiguous genitalia

Molecular biological advances have afforded new techniques for identifying genetic abnormalities. These techniques include Southern blotting, restriction fragment length polymorphisms (RFLP) and polymerase chain reaction (PCR). Such techniques have made it possible to diagnose genetic disease, clone genes, offer prenatal diagnosis and perform genetic engineering (replace missing or defective genes with normal genes).

Diagnostic Modalities

Prenatal diagnostic techniques include:
Ultrasonography
Amniocentesis
Chorionic villus sampling
Alpha-fetoprotein analysis
- ↑ in twins, neural tube defects, GI obstruction, congenital nephrosis, impending fetal demise
- ↓ in Trisomy 21
DNA analysis and enzyme assays

Diseases

Representative Autosomal Dominant Diseases

Achondroplasia
Familial hypercholesterolemia
Gilbert disease
Hereditary hemorrhagic telangiectasis
 (Osler-Weber-Rendu disease)
Huntington disease
Marfan syndrome

Myotonic dystrophy
Neurofibromatosis
Osteogenesis imperfecta, type I
Peutz-Jeghers syndrome
Protein C deficiency
Tuberous sclerosis
von Willebrand disease

Representative Autosomal Recessive Diseases

Alpha-1-antitrypsin deficiency
Congenital adrenal hyperplasia
Cystic fibrosis
Galactosemia
Gaucher disease
Glycogen storage diseases
Homocystinuria

Mucopolysaccharidoses
 (except Hunter disease)
Phenylketonuria (PKU)
Sickle cell anemia
Tay-Sachs disease
Wilson disease

Representative X-linked Disease

Bruton agammaglobulinemia
Color blindness
Duchenne muscular dystrophy
Familial hypophosphatemic rickets
Fragile X syndrome

Hemophilia
Hunter syndrome
Lesch-Nyhan syndrome
Testicular feminization

Sex Chromosome Disorders

Turner syndrome [female, single X chromosome (XO)]
Klinefelter syndrome [male, extra X chromosome (XXY)]

Metabolic Disease

Disease Profiles

Inborn Error of Metabolism
Etiology
The disease of the "inborn errors of metabolism" are primarily caused by either deficiency of an enzyme or failure of enzymatic function which leads to accumulation of a precursor and deficiency of the end product in a metabolic pathway.
Pathophysiologic Abnormality
Abnormalities result from either toxicity of the excessive precursor or harmful effects from the absent product. The placental exchange of metabolic waste products between mother and fetus contributes to a normal infant at birth.
Predisposing Conditions
Most of these diseases are inherited as autosomal recessive conditions.
Symptoms
Presentation is often of a clinically deteriorating neonate who had been previously normal. The clinical picture is similar to that of neonatal sepsis. Symptoms occur during the first week of life and include: poor feeding, vomiting, tachypnea, CNS depression (lethargy, hypotonia and often seizures).
Laboratory Findings
Hypoglycemia, metabolic acidosis, hyperammonemia, ketonuria, liver dysfunction
Potential Complications
Death, mental retardation, failure to thrive
Diagnostic Plan
Neonatal screening programs screen for the following:

Phenylketonuria (PKU)
Galactosemia
Homocystinuria
Hereditary fructose intolerance
Maple syrup urine disease (MSUD)
Tyrosinemia

Initial laboratory evaluation includes:

Arterial blood gas for pH and pCO_2, glucose, ammonia, liver functions, urinalysis for reducing substances

Differential:

High ammonia, nl. pH →→ think urea cycle defects

High ammonia, acidosis →→ think organic acidemias

Nl. ammonia →→ think aminoacidopathies

Urine screening tests include: ferric chloride, nitroprusside & dinitrophenylhydrazine tests

Diagnostic testing includes: urine metabolic screening, urine & serum for amino & organic acids and specific enzyme assays from blood &/or fibroblasts

Therapeutic Plan

Restriction of dietary protein, administration of IV glucose, occ. supplementation of specific vitamin or cofactor

Prognosis

Depends on specific disorder

Endocrinology

Diagnostic Modalities

Hormonal Assays:

Radioimmunoassay

ELISA

Hemoglobin A_{1C} - measurement of glycosylated hemoglobin, an indicator of the prevailing glucose concentration in the blood over the previous 2-3 months. Normal levels are <7%, levels >10-12% indicate poor control in diabetics.

Lipoprotein electrophoresis - electrophoretic separation of the major classes of lipoproteins into:

Chylomicrons

Low density lipoproteins (LDL)

Very low-density lipoproteins (VLDL)

High density lipoproteins (HDL)

Imaging studies:

Bone age

Ultrasound

CT/MRI

Bone scan

Stimulation testing - administration of a substance (usu. a hypothalamic or pituitary hormone) to stimulate a target organ to secrete its hormone (eg, administration of ACTH to stimulate the adrenal glands to secrete cortisol = Cortrosyn stimulation test)

Pathophysiologic Manifestations

Often a hormonal deficiency or excess may lead to a number of clinical or biochemical findings which may include one or more of the following:

Electrolyte abnormalities

Abnormalities of water balance

Aberrations of growth &/or puberty

Other organ system involvement (eye, skin, heart, bone, nervous system)

Disease Profiles

Adrenal Disorders

Congenital Adrenal Hyperplasia

Alternate Terminology

Adrenogenital syndrome

Etiology

Family of autosomal recessive disorders in which there is a deficiency of one of the enzymes necessary for cortisol synthesis. 21-hydroxylase deficiency accounts for >90% of cases.

Pathophysiologic Abnormality

Cortisol and aldosterone deficiencies with accumulation of steroid precursors and excessive androgen production.

Predisposing Conditions

Genetically inherited

Symptoms

Adrenal insufficiency with vomiting, dehydration and shock in first 1 to 4 weeks of life. Signs of early puberty (adrenarche) if late-onset.

Physical Findings

Ambiguous genitalia in female infants. Hyperpigmentation, especially of areolae and scrotum. In older children, pubic hair, body odor, acne, rapid growth, clitoromegaly.

Laboratory Findings

Hyponatremia, hyperkalemia, metabolic acidosis, hypoglycemia, elevated steroid precursors (17-hydroxyprogesterone, deoxycorticosterone), elevated plasma renin activity.

Potential Complications

Death from adrenal insufficiency. In older females, hirsutism and menstrual irregularities.

Differential Diagnosis

Sepsis, GI obstruction (pyloric stenosis), other causes of genital ambiguity

Diagnostic Plan

Electrolytes, steroid precursors, cortisol, plasma renin activity

Therapeutic Plan

Cortisol replacement (10-20 mg/m^2/d), mineralocorticoid replacement (Florinef), IV NS.

Prognosis

Good if appropriate treatment initiated. Potential complication of treatment is iatrogenic Cushings.

Adrenal Insufficiency

Alternate Terminology

Addison's disease

Etiology

Infectious, infiltrative or autoimmune destruction of the adrenal gland

Pathophysiologic Abnormality

Destruction of gland usually leads to both glucocorticoid and mineralocorticoid deficiencies

Predisposing Condition

Autoimmune polyglandular syndrome, tumors or anomalies of the CNS, genetically inherited forms such as CAH & adrenoleukodystrophy

Symptoms

Nausea, vomiting, fatigue, anorexia, weight loss

Laboratory Findings

Hyponatremia, hyperkalemia, hypocortisolism, hypoglycemia

Potential Complications

Death

Differential Diagnosis

Primary causes: Autoimmune (most common), CAH, fungal infiltration (TB, sarcoid, histoplasmosis), bilateral hemorrhage (Waterhouse-Friderichsen), adrenoleukodystrophy

Secondary causes: hypothalamic/pituitary defects, anorexia nervosa, iatrogenic

Diagnostic Plan

ACTH stimulation test for cortisol response; normal response should be >15 ug/dl

Therapeutic Plan

Cortisol & mineralocorticoid replacement. Acutely, IV NS & Solu-cortef

Prognosis

Good. Need additional hydrocortisone during times of stress (illness, surgery, etc)

Thyroid Disorders

Hyperthyroidism/Graves' Disease

Alternative Terminology

Thyrotoxicosis

Etiology

Autoimmune, association with thyrotropin receptor antibodies, ie, thyroid stimulating immunoglobulins (TSI), long-acting thyroid stimulator (LATS) and thyrotropin binding inhibitor immunoglobulin (TBII). Genetic predisposition with HLA-B8 & -DR3 association.

Pathophysiologic Abnormality

Defect in T lymphocyte suppressor cell function resulting in production of TSI and hyperthyroidism.

Predisposing Conditions

Genetic predisposition and environmental triggers. Female preponderance 6:1.

Symptoms

Nervousness, increased appetite with weight loss, heat intolerance, palpitations, hyperactivity, increased sweating, sleep disturbance, drop in school performance.

Physical Findings

Goiter, tachycardia, widened pulse pressure, tremor, exophthalmos, thyroid bruit, eyelid lag.

Laboratory Findings

Elevated T_4, Free T_4 & T_3RU, suppressed TSH, TSI or TBII positive in >90%. Radioiodine scan demonstrates high uptake.

Potential Complications

Hypertension, cardiac arrhythmias, thyroid storm, progressive ophthalmopathy

Differential Diagnosis

Hashitoxicosis, thyroiditis, autonomously functioning nodule, thyroid hormone resistance.

Diagnostic Plan

Thyroid function tests, thyroid antibodies. Scan not routinely necessary.

Therapeutic Plan

Three options:

• antithyroid drug therapy (propylthiouracil (PTU) and methimazole) (propanolol used as an adjunct to treat symptoms)

• radioiodine therapy

• surgery

Prognosis

Disease can be controlled but not cured. Risk of relapse highest with medical treatment (3-40%). Risk of hypothyroidism with radioiodine. Drug toxicities include agranulocytosis, arthritis, hepatitis and glomerulonephritis. Surgical complications include hypoparathyroidism and hypocalcemia.

Acquired Hypothyroidism

Alternate Terminology

Hashimoto's thyroiditis

Etiology

Autoimmune; overtreatment of hyperthyroidism

Pathophysiologic Abnormality

Production of antithyroid antibodies - antithyroglobulin and antimicrosomal antibodies in autoimmune disease

Predisposing Conditions

Female preponderance; genetic predisposition

Symptoms

Lethargy, weight gain, cold intolerance, dry skin and hair, constipation, delayed puberty, poor growth

Physical Findings

Dull appearance, dry skin and hair, delay in relaxation phase of deep tendon reflexes, puffiness

Laboratory Findings

Elevated TSH, low T_4, Free T_4 & T_3RU, positive antibodies in autoimmune disease

Potential Complications

Myxedema, myocardial dysfunction

Differential Diagnosis

Chronic lymphocytic thyroiditis, TRH/TSH deficiency, iatrogenic (antithyroid therapy or post-irradiation)

Diagnostic Plan

Thyroid function tests and antithyroid antibodies

Therapeutic Plan

Replacement with L-thyroxine (100 μcg/m^2)

Prognosis

Excellent on replacement

Congenital Hypothyroidism

Alternate Terminology

Cretinism

Etiology

Lack of appropriate development of fetal thyroid gland, exposure to maternal antithyroid agents, TRH/TSH deficiency, enzymatic defects

Pathophysiologic Abnormality

Thyroid dysgenesis (aplasia, hypoplasia, ectopy) results in lack of thyroid hormone production

Predisposing Conditions

Exposure to maternal antithyroid agents

Symptoms

Poor feeding, lethargy, prolonged jaundice, constipation, hoarse cry, developmental delay

Physical Findings

Dull, coarse facies, enlarged tongue, large fontanelles, hypotonia, umbilical hernia

Laboratory Findings

Elevated TSH, low-normal T$_4$, FreeT$_4$, low T$_3$RU (newborn screening program tests T$_4$ and TSH), delayed bone age

Potential Complications

Mental and growth retardation if untreated

Diagnostic Plan

Thyroid function tests, thyroid scan; TSH is high in primary hypothyroidism and low in central hypothyroidism

Therapeutic Plan

Replacement with L-thyroxine (100 ucg/m^2/d)

Prognosis

Good with early treatment (by 4-6 weeks of age)

Insulin-Dependent Diabetes Mellitus, Type I

Etiology

(Most common endocrine/metabolic disease of childhood) Autoimmune with contributing genetic and environmental factors

Pathophysiologic Abnormality

Autoimmune-mediated destruction of insulin-producing pancreatic *B* cells. Islet cell antibodies and insulin autoantibodies present months to years prior to symptoms.

Predisposing Conditions

HLA-association (DR3/DR4); absence of aspartic acid at position 57 of the DQ *B* chain

Symptoms

Polyphagia, polydipsia, polyuria, weight loss

Physical Findings

Weight loss

Laboratory Findings

Hyperglycemia (random blood glucose >200 mg/dl diagnostic) glycosuria

Potential Complications

Diabetic ketoacidosis

Diagnostic Plan

Blood chemistries, glucose tolerance test

Therapeutic Plan

Insulin replacement

Prognosis

Long-term complications include retinopathy, nephropathy, neuropathy, heart disease

Diabetic Ketoacidosis

Pathophysiologic Abnormality

Insulin deficiency results in increased glucose production, decreased glucose utilization, increase in counterregulatory hormones including epinephrine, growth hormone, cortisol and glucagon with resultant lipolysis, fatty acid mobilization and ketoacid production

Predisposing Conditions

Infection, stress, inadequate insulin administration

Symptoms

Polyuria, polydipsia, nausea, vomiting, abdominal pain

Physical Findings

Dehydration, deep, rapid (Kussmaul) respirations, acetone odor to breath

Laboratory Findings

Hyperglycemia, acidosis, ketosis, ketonuria, hyponatremia (dilutional), elevated BUN, decreased bicarbonate

Potential Complications

Death, cerebral edema during correction

Diagnostic Plan

Serum electrolytes, glucose, ketones, pH, urine ketones

Therapeutic Plan

IVF with NS to correct dehydration & acidosis, insulin & potassium administration, sodium bicarbonate not given unless pH <7.1, IV glucose not given until BS $\leq$ 300

Calcium/Vitamin D Disorders

Rickets -

Etiology

Deficiency of or lack of response to vitamin D or phosphorous

Pathophysiologic Abnormality

Abnormalities of mineral availability and excessive bone resorption lead to decrease in bone mass (osteopenia) and inadequate bone mineralization

Predisposing Conditions

Low birth weight/prematurity; exclusively breast-fed; anticonvulsant drugs; malabsorption; chronic renal disease

Symptoms

Bowing of lower extremities, pain with weight-bearing, fractures

Physical Findings

Bowed legs, widened wrists, "rachitic rosary" (beading of ribs)

Laboratory Findings/Differential Diagnosis

Increased alkaline phosphate in all forms

Diagnosis	Calcium	Phos.	25,OHD3	1,25(OH)$_2$D3
Vit. D. Deficiency 1,25 hydroxylase deficiency	low-nl	low-nl	low	variable
(Vit. D dep. type I) Vit. D resistant	low	low-nl	high	low
-(Vit. D receptor defect)	low	low-nl	nl-high	high
Familial hypophosphatemic rickets (most common form in USA)	normal	low	high	low

Potential Complications
> Fractures, poor growth, nephrocalcinosis secondary to treatment

Diagnostic Plan
> Serum & urine calcium & phosphorous, vitamin D metabolites, alkaline phosphatase, electrolytes, X-rays

Therapeutic Plan
> Vitamin D & phosphorous supplementation for familial hypophosphatemic form; 1,25(OH)2D3 alone for Vit. dependent and Vit. D resistant forms

Pubertal Disorders

Normal Puberty
Controlled by CNS maturation, hypothalamic secretion of gonadotropin-releasing hormone (GnRH or LHRH) stimulates pituitary secretion of gonadotropins, LH (luteinizing hormone) and FSH (follicle stimulating hormone) that act on the ovaries to produce estrogen and the testes to produce testosterone. Pubertal onset signaled by breast development in females and testicular enlargement (≥2.5 cm) in males.

Definition of Terms

Thelarche - breast development
> **Adrenarche** - adrenal androgen production leading to secondary sexual characteristics (axillary & pubic hair, acne)
> **Menarche** - initiation of menses

Delayed Puberty
Definition
> Lack of pubertal signs by age 13 years in females and 14 years in males
Etiology
> Lack of sex steroid production from gonads or lack of input from hypothalamus or pituitary
Predisposing Conditions
> CNS anomalies/tumors, autoimmune/postinfectious destruction of gonads, iatrogenic (s/p chemotherapy or irradiation) chronic illness, malnutrition, chromosomal abnormalities
Physical Findings
> Lack of breast budding or testicular enlargement, physical features of specific syndrome (eg, Turner syndrome), anosmia (Kallman syndrome)
Laboratory Findings
> Primary gonadal failure: high gonadotropins, low sex steroids
> Hypothalamic/pituitary causes: low gonadotropins, low sex steroids
Potential Complications
> Many causes also lead to sterility
Diagnostic Plan
> Sex steroid levels, LHRH stimulation test to assess gonadotropin production, thyroid function, rule out chronic disease, bone age, karyotype
Therapeutic Plan
> Estrogen or testosterone replacement

Precocious Puberty
Definition
> Pubertal onset <8 years in females, <9 years in males
Etiology
> CNS lesions, gonadal tumors, adrenal disorders (CAH, tumors), exogenous sex steroids
Pathophysiologic Abnormality
> Premature activation of hypothalamic-pituitary-gonadal axis or autonomous production of sex steroids leading to development of sexual characteristics

Predisposing Conditions

CNS tumors/anomalies, hydrocephalus, CAH

Physical Findings

Breast development, testicular enlargement, rapid growth, secondary sexual characteristics

Laboratory Findings

Central (CNS) causes:	high gonadotropins, high sex steroids
Peripheral causes:	low gonadotropins, high sex steroids

Advanced bone age, elevated steroid precursors in CAH

Potential Complications

Early epiphyseal closure with short stature, psychological distress

Diagnostic Plan

Bone age, pelvic/testicular/adrenal ultrasound, head MRI, gonadotropins in response to LHRH stimulation, adrenal precursors, sex steroid levels

Therapeutic Plan

Appropriate to etiology, ie, tumor removal, glucocorticoids for CAH, etc, GnRH agonist (Depo-lupron) for central causes to suppress gonadotropin secretion

Prognosis

Depends on etiology

Darin Brannan
A Eugene Osburn
Jane E Puls

Developmental Considerations

Host Defense

A host defense system helps ensure the homeostasis of the human organism by providing protection against infection, malignancy and autoimmune diseases. Some of the defense system is static, such as the skin barrier and mobile cilia. Others are able to adapt to challenges presented to the organism as "foreign substances". The major components of the adaptive system of defense are the T lymphocytes, B lymphocytes, phagocytes and the complement system.

Host defense can be subdivided into nonspecific and specific components. The nonspecific defense mechanisms include skin and mucosal barriers, complement system, phagocytic system, and normal intestinal flora (impeding bacterial or yeast overgrowth). Specific defense mechanisms are antibody-mediated immunity and cell-mediated immunity.

Undifferentiated stem cells in the fetal bone marrow and liver give rise to three cell lines, which differentiate according to the microenvironment in which they mature. Stem cells which migrate to the thymus and develop under the influence of local humoral factors become T-Cells. Those which migrate to the bone marrow become B-Cells and enter the circulation to populate lymphoid follicles.

B-Cells

B-Cells differentiate into plasma cells which secrete immunoglobulins. The classes of and function of immunoglobulins are:

IgM   -   Adult levels are produced by 1 year of age
      -   10% of immunoglobulin pool
      -   Forms rapidly after antigenic stimulation
      -   Aids in opsonization and agglutination

IgG   -   Adult levels are produced by 5-7 years of age
      -   70-75% of immunoglobulin pool
      -   Protect against bacteria, viruses and fungi
      -   Major antibody of rechallenge immune responses
      -   Persists after antigenic stimulation
      -   Crosses placenta in latter half of 3rd trimester

IgA	-	Adult levels are produced by 10-14 years of age
	-	15-20% of immunoglobulin pool
	-	Secretory antibody in saliva, lacrimal fluid and colostrum, nasal secretions, bronchial secretions and intestinal secretions
IgD	-	Less than 1% of immunoglobulin pool
	-	Serves as receptor site on circulating B cells
IgE	-	Small amount of immunoglobulin pool
	-	Found on surface of mast cells and basophils
	-	Allergic individuals often have high serum levels

T-Cells

T-Cells function as regulators and amplifiers of the immunologic response of other immunocompetent cells. They release soluble mediators (lymphokines) in response to appropriate antigenic challenge which in turn recruit macrophages, granulocytes and other immunocompetent cells. Some of the T-Cells are cytotoxic cells and can lyse target cells selectively. Helper T-Cells have a surface antigen marker termed CD4 and suppressor (cytotoxic) T-Cells have a CD8 surface antigen.

Phagocytes

Phagocytes are able to migrate toward a chemical stimulus initiated by an inflammatory response, ingest and then destroy engulfed microorganisms. Mast cells and basophils are mediators of the immediate hypersensitivity response. They have receptors with a high affinity to IgE but can be activated by non IgE mechanisms as well. Upon activation, they secrete mediators of an inflammatory response within seconds, the most prominent being histamine.

Complement System

Components of the complement system are involved in the inflammatory response in both effector and regulatory functions. There are two pathways of complement activation: the classic and the alternative. Either leads to activation of a common final pathway, which results in the formation of a membrane attack complex. The classic pathway is initiated by IgG or IgM antigen-antibody complexes; the alternative pathway does not require antibody for its activation. C3 is consumed as the first component of either pathway. Regulatory proteins modulate the activity of complement. Alternative pathway activation occurs only as a result of loss of inhibition mediated by these regulatory proteins. Most bacteria cells lack activators of these inhibitors. However, bacteria rich in sialic acid - such as group B *Streptococcus, Neisseria* and *E coli* - are able to resist alternative pathway activation and therefore are more pathogenic in individuals who lack sufficient antibody activators of the classic pathway (eg, neonates).

Diagnostic Modalities

History

       Growth deficiency

       Chronic infections

       Recurrent infections (more than expected given infant or child's home situation (only child, day care, etc))

       Skin rash(es)

       Infected by opportunistic organisms

       Continual infections (without periods of good health between)

       Infected with microbial agents of normally low pathogenicity

Physical Examination

       Ht, Wt

       General appearance, energy level, (pale? apathetic? irritable?)

       Skin rashes (eczema, abcesses)

       Mucous membranes (*Candida*)

       Lymph nodes, tonsils (hyper or hypo trophic)

       Hepatosplenomegaly

       Ataxia

       Developmental abilities

Laboratory Data

    Screening Tests

- General
  * CBC with differential
  * X-rays, bone scans to identify infections
  * Cultures as indicated
  * Erythrocyte sedimentation rate
- Tests of antibody-mediated (humoral: B-Cell) immunity
  * Quantitative immunoglobulin levels of IgG, IgM, IgA, IgE
  * Isohemagglutinin titer (anti-A, anti-B) to measure IgM function
  * Patient's antibody response to immunization to diphtheria, tetanus toxoid and measles-mumps-rubella vaccine
- Tests of cell-mediated (T-Cell) immunity
  * Absolute lymphocyte count
  * Delayed hypersensitivity skin test to *Candida*, tetanus toxoid, tuberculin and antigen to mumps

- Tests of phagocytosis-mediated immunity
  * Absolute neutrophil count
  * Nitroblue tetrazolium (NBT) dye test to measure neutrophil metabolic function
  * IgE level
- Tests of complement-mediated immunity
  * Total hemolytic complement (CH50) to measure complement activity
  * C3, C4 levels to measure important pathway components

Advanced Immunologic Tests

- Antibody-mediated
  * HIV antibody
  * B-Cell quantitation
  * IgG subclasses
  * Secretory antibody levels
  * Pre-existing antibody levels: measles, polio, diphtheria, tetanus
  * Specific antibody response: *S pneumoniae, H influenzae*
- Cell-mediated
  * T-Cell quantitation and subpopulations
  * Mitogen stimulation response
  * Mixed lymphocyte culture assays
  * Thymic hormone assays
- Phagocyte-mediated
  * Rebuck skin window for chemotaxis
  * Chemotaxis, adhesion, aggregation assays
  * Enzyme assays: myeloperoxidase
  * Metabolic assays: chemiluminescence
  * Phagocytic and bactericidal assays
- Complement-mediated
  * Classic pathway individual component assays
  * Alternative pathway individual component assays
  * C1 esterase inhibitor
  * Chemotactic factors
  * Opsonic assays

Pathophysiologic Manifestations

Clinical Characteristics of B-Cell Defects
- Recurrent pyrogenic infections with extracellular encapsulated organisms (eg, *S pneumoniae, H influenzae*)
- Otitis, sinusitis, recurrent pneumonia, bronchiectasis, conjunctivitis
- Diarrhea, especially due to *Giardia lamblia* infection
- Decreased serum immunoglobulins
- Growth is usually normal
- Increased rate of viral and fungal infections are rare (except for enterovirus encephalitis and poliomyelitis)

Prognosis
Survival to adulthood, or years after onset

Clinical Characteristics of T-Cell Defects
- Recurrent infections with opportunistic or less virulent organisms (eg, viruses, fungi, protozoa, mycobacteria)
- Malabsorption, diarrhea, growth retardation, failure to thrive
- Anergy
- Graft-versus-host reaction if given non-irradiated blood
- Live virus vaccinations or BCG vaccinations can be fatal
- High incidence of malignance

Prognosis
Survival beyond infancy or childhood is rare; improving with better treatments

Clinical Characteristics of Phagocytic Defects
- Recurrent skin infections with bacteria and fungi (eg, *Staphylococcus, Pseudomonas, E coli,* and *Aspergillus*)
- Abscesses of lymph nodes, subcutaneous tissue, liver and lung (pulmonary infections are common and contribute to chronic lung disease)
- Bone and joint infections are common

Clinical Characteristics of Complement Defects
- Recurrent bacterial infections with extracellular pyogenic organisms (eg, *S pneumoniae, H influenzae*)
- Unusual susceptibility to recurrent *Neisseria* infections (eg, *Gonococcus* and *Meningococcus*)
- Increased incidence of autoimmune disease (eg, SLE, rheumatoid arthritis, sarcoidosis)
- Recurrent or severe skin and respiratory tract infections

Disease Profiles

Pediatric Acquired Immunodeficiency Syndrome
    Alternate Terminology
        AIDS
    Etiology
        Infection with the human immunodeficiency virus, type 1 (HIV-1)
    Pathophysiology
        Depletion of CD4 cells, anergy, poor antibody response to de novo antigens, hypergammaglobulinemia.
    Predisposing Conditions
        Vertical transmission (transplacental, perinatal, breast feeding), blood inoculation, sexual abuse, sexual activity, injecting drug use. Any condition that allows exposure to HIV-positive body fluids.
    Symptoms
        History suggests child is at risk, recurrent infections, poor growth, infected with opportunistic organisms.
    Physical Findings
        Hepatosplenomegaly, lymphadenopathy, growth failure, candidiasis, diarrhea.
    Laboratory Findings
        Antibody testing for diagnosis (remember that infants may have persistent maternal IgG anti-HIV for up to 15 months. The presence of IgA anti-HIV represents specific production by the infant.)
    Differential Diagnosis
        Severe Combined Immunodeficiency (SCID), hypogammaglobulinemia
    Potential Complications
        Infections with encapsulated organisms, gram-negative bacteria, opportunistic organism, etc; continued poor growth; death.
    Therapeutic Plan
        Treatment of specific infections, infection prophylaxis and anti-retroviral therapy.

Selected Primary Immunodeficiency Disorders

DISORDER	CLINICAL MANIFESTATIONS	INHERITANCE
B-Cell (antibody-mediated)		
X-linked agammaglobulinemia (Bruton's)	Recurrent pyogenic infections of the CNS,0 sinuses, middle ear, lungs and skin	Xq22
Dysgammaglobulinemia IgA deficiency IgM deficiency IgG subclass of deficiency	Recurrent infections of sinuses, lungs; gastrointestinal disease	Variable AR Gene deletion
Common variable immunodeficiency	Infections of sinuses, middle ear, lungs; giardiasis; malabsorption; autoimmune disease	AR, AD
Transcobalamin II deficiency	Recurrent infections; megaloblastic anemia; intestinal villous atrophy; defective granulocytic bactericidal activity	AD
T-Cell (cell-mediated)		
Wiskott-Aldrich syndrome	Eczema; thrombocytopenia; recurrent infections; malignancy	X-linked
DiGeorge syndrome	Hypoparathyroidism; facial abnormalities; cardiac anomalies	90% have 22 q11 deletion
Ataxia-telangiectasia	Oculocutaneous telangiectasia; progressive cerebellar ataxia; bronchiectasis; malignancy	AR
Severe combined immunodeficiency	Recurrent infections; chronic diarrhea; failure to thrive	X-linked, AR
Complement		
Hereditary angioedema (C1 esterase inhibitor deficiency)	Recurrent facial, laryngeal, GI or limb edema	AD
Neutrophil		
Hyper IgE (Job) syndrome	Recurrent staphylococcal skin abscesses, chronic eczema, and otitis media; severe periodontal disease	Unknown
Chronic granulomatous disease	Suppurative lymphadenitis, hepatosplenomegaly, pneumonitis, osteomyelitis	X-linked and autosomal

Secondary Immunodeficiency Disorders

Many diseases interfere temporarily or permanently with the function of the normal immune system. The two most common significant diseases to do this day are HIV and protein-calorie malnutrition. Others are listed below. Diagnosis and treatment are dependent on the specific etiology.

Causes of Secondary Immunodeficiencies

- **Premature and newborn infants**
- **Infections**
  Bacterial, viral (HIV, CMV, measles, rubella, hepatitis, Epstein-Barr virus), fungal, tuberculosis, malaria
- **Chronic Disease**
  Sickle-cell disease (functional splenectomy), Cystic fibrosis
- **Neoplastic Disease**
  Leukemia, Hodgkin's disease, nonlymphoid cancer
- **Surgery and Trauma**
  Burns, splenectomy, stress
- **Autoimmune Disease**
  SLE, Rheumatoid arthritis, graft-versus-host disease
- **Protein-Losing States**
  Protein losing-enteropathy, nephrotic syndrome
- **Immunosuppressive Treatment**
  Chemotherapy, radiation therapy, corticosteroids
- **Hereditary and Metabolic Diseases**
  Malnutrition, uremia, diabetes mellitus, sickle-cell anemia, chromosomal abnormalities

Hypersensitivity Reactions

Mechanisms which provide host defense can also cause tissue damage if the reaction is exaggerated. Four major types of reaction are recognized:

Type I
- anaphylactic, atopic or reaginic reaction
- mediated by IgE triggered release of histamine and other substances (eg, hay fever, extrinsic asthma, anaphylactic shock)

Type II
- antibody-mediated cytotoxic reaction
- IgG or IgM binds to cell-carried antigens resulting in lysis (eg, autoimmune hemolytic anemia)

Type III
- Immune-complex mediated reaction with tissue deposition
- complement activation is involved (eg, autoimmune diseases, serum sickness, Arthus reactions)

Type IV
- Sensitized T-Cells bind to cellular antigens and result in lysis (eg, Graft rejection, contact dermatitis)

Autoimmune Diseases

Autoimmune diseases arise in situations where the host defense mechanisms recognize the individuals own cell antigens as foreign. The most common mediators of autoimmune diseases are misdirected Type I and Type III hypersensitivity reactions. Some of the conditions that occur when the system goes awry are:
Systemic lupus erythematosus
Rheumatoid arthritis
Rheumatic fever
Serum sickness
Mucocutaneous lymph node syndrome (Kawasaki disease)
Henoch-Schönlein purpura
Atopic dermatitis/Eczema
Lyme disease

Diane Kittredge

Developmental Considerations

Childhood cancers are rare events but important to recognize because of excellent treatment outcomes for many of the cancers, if found early. Cancer is the second leading killer of children between ages 1-14 (injuries are first), causing 10% of deaths in this age group. One out of 600 children will be diagnosed with cancer sometime in the first 15 years of life. Childhood cancer comprises only 1% of all cancers, but if children with cancer do not survive they have many years of "lost life".

Childhood cancers are quite distinct from adult cancers. The most common types, in order of frequency, are:

Leukemia
Central nervous system tumors
Lymphoma
Neuroblastoma
Soft tissue sarcoma
Wilms' tumor
Bone tumors
Retinoblastoma
Others

Half of childhood cancers are due to leukemia and central nervous system (CNS) tumors.

Most cancers in children are still of unknown etiology. The postulated candidates for causing a malignant transformation in normal cell lines are similar to those postulated for birth defects involving structural or metabolic derangements:

Genetic propensities
Environmental agents
Altered immunogenicity
Some viral infections

Certain cancers have a predilection for special age groups:
    Neuroblastoma (tumor of neural crest origin) -- infants
    Wilms' tumor (renal tumor) -- infants
    Retinoblastoma (in retina, presents as white pupil) -- infants
    Acute lymphocytic leukemia (ALL) -- preschoolers
    Osteosarcoma (usually in long bones) -- in growing teens
Certain cancers are related to a genetic defect:
    Retinoblastoma in families with dominant gene defect
    Leukemia in children with Trisomy 21
    Hepatoma (liver tumor) in children with certain metabolic defects of the liver
    Skin cancer (during childhood) in children with albinism
    Diverse tumors in congenital syndromes with disorders of genetic repair mechanisms

Diagnostic Modalities

The diagnostic workup depends on the type of cancer suspected. Even though childhood cancer is a rare event, cancer is in the differential diagnosis for many common childhood symptom complexes (see pathophysiologic manifestations below).

Be on the alert for symptoms and signs of cancer.

Take time to listen to the parent who senses something is seriously out of the ordinary for his/her child.

Be complete on all routine physical examinations, especially noting growth curves, head growth (0-18 months), eye findings, abdominal masses, lymph nodes, and skin lesions.

For any persistent, unexplained illness or weight loss do screening laboratory.

101

Regardless of the type of cancer suspected, it will be essential to obtain a confirmatory tissue diagnosis. This is best done in a referral center which specializes in pediatric cancer treatment. This step involves, depending on the type of cancer:

Cell morphology
Cytogenetics
Immunotyping
Disease staging (extent of primary tumor and metastasis)

Pathophysiologic Considerations

SIGNS AND SYMPTOMS SUGGESTIVE OF CANCER

Prolonged fever
Night sweats
Weight loss
Abdominal masses
Thoracic masses
Painless lymphadenopathy
Bone pain
Petechiae
Signs of increased intracranial pressure
Ataxia
Exophthalmos
Proptosis
Leukokoria
Moles which are changing

Common Clinical Presentations for Childhood Neoplasms

Consider neoplasm in the differential diagnosis of the following common pediatric signs and symptoms:

Abnormal CBC
* anemia associated with depression of at least one other cell line
* extreme leukocytosis
* neutropenia
* low platelets plus anemia or abnormal WBC

    Most Common Neoplasms
    leukemia, or solid tumor with bone marrow invasion

    Evaluation
    bone marrow

Abdominal Mass
* in infancy or early childhood, with or without other findings

    Most Common Neoplasms
    neuroblastomas, Wilms' tumor

    Evaluation
    ultrasound to define renal system, liver, spleen (may also need CT to define mass

Adenopathy
* large non-tender nodes in the head and neck region which fail to respond to antibiotics
* generalized adenopathy, associated with constitutional symptoms and/or depressed blood counts

    Most Common Neoplasms
    leukemia, Hodgkin's lymphoma; also consider HIV/AIDS

    Evaluation
    CBC, node biopsy; consider bone marrow

White Pupil
* in infancy and early childhood

    Most Common Neoplasms
    retinoblastoma (can be hereditary)

    Evaluation
    urgent referral to ophthalmologist

Limb Pain
- unexplained limp, bone pain, or arthralgias
  Most Common Neoplasms
  > leukemia (any age), primary bone tumor (especially in growing teenager)
  Evaluation
  > X-ray and CBC

Headache
- persistent severe headache worsening over time in spite of standard therapy (especially with vomiting or focal CNS findings)
- persistent headache in children under 4 years of age
- headaches which are worse in the morning and which awaken the child from sleep
  Most Common Neoplasms
  > primary CNS tumors (small tumors blocking flow of CSF or large space occupying lesions in the cerebellum or lateral hemispheres)
  Evaluation
  > careful funduscopic exam to assess optic disc; imaging study of CNS (consult with specialist about best study for each clinical situation)

Seizures
- focal seizures, after the newborn period
- generalized seizures with focal neurologic exam
  Most Common Neoplasms
  > primary CNS tumors (see, Headache, above)
  Evaluation
  > EEG and imaging study of the CNS (consult with specialist about best study for each clinical situation)

Emergencies in Children with Cancer

Fever and Neutropenia ($\leq 500/mm^3$)
  Comment
  > seen in bone marrow invasion and as sequela of therapy; these children should be considered septic until proved otherwise

Do

> prompt history and exam; obtain cultures; start empiric broad spectrum parenteral antibiotics

Chickenpox Exposure or Illness
Comment

> varicella illness is very severe in a child who is immune suppressed due to cancer or its treatment

Do

> give varicella zoster immunoglobulin within 72 hours of exposure; intravenous antiviral therapy after 72 hours

Rapidly Increasing Intracranial Pressure
Comment

> seen in leukemic infiltration of the CNS and CNS tumors blocking CSF flow

Do

> emergency care to reduce pressure; urgent referral for radiation or other treatment

Hyperleukocytosis (WBC > 100,000/mm^3)
Comment

> seen in AML, and T-Cell ALL; these children are at risk for complications from vascular occlusion, especially cerebral vascular accidents

Do

> IV hydration, consult hematologist urgently

Late, Long Term Complications of Cancer in Childhood

Endocrine suppression (growth, thyroid, delayed puberty)
Learning problems (if CNS irradiation done for first tumor)
Reproductive failure
Second tumors

Therapeutic Options

In 1940 only 5% of children with cancer survived. In 1990 the survival rate had risen to 65%.

Treatment depends on definitive tissue diagnosis, best done in a referral center where sophisticated morphology, cytogenetics and immunotyping can be done. Multicenter treatment protocols are the norm in pediatric cancer treatment, since the diseases are so infrequent and the science is advancing so rapidly. In the last few decades, remarkable improvements in outcome have been achieved. For most of the common cancer in childhood, more than 50% of children can expect long-term survival and cure.

Surgery, radiation treatment, chemotherapy, and bone marrow transplant may be used, depending on the characteristics of the tumor. Psychosocial support to the child and family is essential, as is rehabilitation and educational planning.

Disease Profiles

Leukemia
    Etiology
        Classification
            Acute (97% of childhood leukemias)
                Acute lymphocytic leukemia (80% of acute childhood leukemia)
                Acute nonlymphocytic leukemia (17% of acute childhood leukemia)
            Chronic (3% of childhood leukemias)
                All chronic leukemias in childhood are nonlymphocytic
    Pathophysiologic Abnormality
        bone marrow replacement by leukemia cells resulting in anemia, hemorrhagic diathesis, susceptibility to infection and bone pain; reticuloendothelial system infiltration resulting in hepatosplenomegaly and lymphadenopathy

Predisposing Conditions
> immunodeficiency states, solid tumors, congenital bone marrow failure

Symptoms
> pallor, irritability, fatigue, fever, symptoms of infection, bone pain

Physical Findings
> lymphadenopathy, hepatosplenomegaly, petechiae, ecchymosis, signs of infection

Laboratory Findings
> anemia, thrombocytopenia, neutropenia, blast cells in peripheral smear (can be missed by automated cell counters); bone marrow examination; diagnostic cell morphology

Potential Complications
> hyperuricemia, hyperkalemia, complications of anemia, thrombocytopenia, dysfunctional WBCs; tissue infiltration

Diagnostic Plan
> bone marrow aspiration

Therapeutic Plan
> antileukemic therapy dependent on type of leukemia

Prognosis
> Favorable prognostic indicators:
>> age 2-7 years
>> white
>> female
>> initial WBC <10,000
>> normal IgG, IgM, IgA
>> non-T, non-B cell ALL

Central Nervous System Tumors

Second most common form of childhood cancer (20% of total childhood cancers)

Etiology

Classification

> Tumors of Astrocytic Origin
>> high-grade astrocytomas (arise above tentorium)
>> low-grade astrocytomas (arise below the tentorium in the cerebellum)
>> brain stem gliomas

Tumors of Neuroepithelial Origin
medulloblastoma
primitive neuroectodermal tumors

Pathophysiologic Abnormality
mass lesion causing focal neurologic deficits and increased intracranial
pressure

Symptoms
symptoms of increased intracranial pressure; symptoms due to focal
neurologic involvement, eg, headache, vomiting (without diarrhea)

Physical Findings
signs of increased intracranial pressure; focal neurologic deficits; ataxia
and nystagmus if lesion below tentorium

Diagnostic Plan
MRI of head (much more sensitive than CT); CT with contrast material

Therapeutic Plan
surgical resection, chemotherapy and radiation therapy are all used, but all
have potential serious side effects

Neuroblastoma
Second most common solid tumor in childhood (brain tumor is most common solid tumor)

Pathophysiologic Abnormality
malignancy of neural crest cells; signs and symptoms depend on whether
tumor is in the head and neck, chest or abdomen

Predisposing Conditions
infants and preschool children; half are under 2 years of age

Laboratory Findings
elevated vanillymandelic acid (VMA), elevated homovanillic acid (HMA)

Diagnostic Plan
establish staging:

Stage	I	localized
Stage	II	does not cross midline
Stage	III	tumor crosses midline
Stage	IV	metastatic dissemination
Stage	IVS	in young infants with metastasis to skin, liver, bone marrow, but not cortical bone

Therapeutic Plan
surgical resection for Stage I, II and IVS; chemotherapy

Peggy J Hines
A Eugene Osburn

Developmental Considerations

General

Infants under 2 to 3 months of age are not able to isolate and localize infections very effectively. Also, they may not at that age show signs of infection other than temperature changes -- either fever or hypothermia. Therefore, infants under 2 months of age with a rectal temperature over 38.5 C, or who are hypothermic should have a "Sepsis Workup" and be started on IV antibiotics until the culture results indicate it is safe to stop them.

Even if their temperature is less than 38.5 C, infants under 2 months of age who are found to have an infection which is presumably due to a bacterial cause (eg, pneumonia, otitis media, UTI), should be assumed to be incapable of localizing the infection, and started on IV antibiotics after a "Sepsis Workup" is done. For example, the finding of concurrent meningitis requires a longer course of antibiotics than does otitis media alone.

Temperature Regulation and Fever

A child's temperature is normally lower in the early morning than late in the afternoon after they have been active. The maximal daily temperature of children usually occurs between 5:00 and 7:00 PM.

Excessive clothing can interfere with the child's ability to dissipate normal body heat and raise its temperature.

A normal homeostatic mechanism establishes the temperature threshold in children at around 41.1 C (106 F).

Leukocytes have greater phagocytic activity at 38 to 40 C than at lower temperatures.

Fever per se does not cause convulsions. Febrile seizures occur in 5% of children; the seizure occurs during the rise in temperature. Thus, if a child has a high fever for hours or days, he/she will not suddenly have a convulsion because of fever alone. If the underlying cause of the fever is something which irritates the CNS, such as meningitis, then a seizure may occur, but it is the meningitis which causes the convulsion, not the fever.

A decrease in temperature after administration of antipyretics does not distinguish between bacterial and viral infections.

Because of its association with Reye's syndrome in children and adolescents, aspirin should not be used to treat fever in these groups.

There are literally hundreds of diseases which have fever as one of their components. Since there are so many causes of fever, the finding of fever **alone** does not narrow the list of diagnostic possibilities much.

General Causes of Fever
• Infections
• Vaccines
• Drugs
• Collagen-vascular diseases
• Inflammatory diseases
• Endocrine disorders (thyrotoxicosis)
• Malignancy
• High environmental temperatures
• CNS lesions affecting the hypothalamus/brainstem
• Anhydrotic ectodermal dysplasia
• Dehydration
• Strenuous exercise
• Factitious fever

Other Considerations Related to Age

Placentally-transferred maternal immunity lasts a few months. Because it does, it influences when immunizations should be begun in the infant.

Children in day care get more URIs ("colds") for their age than those exposed to fewer contacts. It is unknown to what extent these children are protected from URIs in later school years because of an already acquired immunity to certain viral agents.

There is no such thing as a "viral syndrome". A fever without an obvious cause in a child does not necessarily mean the child has a viral infection.

Diagnostic Modalities

Physical Examination

Region	Focus	Significant Abnormalities
General Appearance	Playfulness	Disinterest in activities or play
	Interactiveness	Withdrawn demeanor
	Alertness	Unaware of those in the room
	Consolability	Unresponsive to comforting
	Irritability with movement	Movement of inflamed tissue, including the meninges, causes pain
	Color	Pallor or Cyanosis
	Hydration	Sunken eyes or fontanel, dry mucous membranes
HEENT	Fontanelle	Bulging or Depressed
	Nuchal rigidity	Brudzenski and Kernig signs
	Rhinorrhea	Purulent discharge may be due to sinusitis
	Tympanic membranes	Erythema, lack of mobility
	Drooling	Found in severe pharyngitis, gingivostomatitis, retropharyngeal abscess, and epiglottitis
Heart	Murmurs	New onset in Rheumatic Fever, endocarditis
	Friction rubs	Suspect pericarditis
	Distant heart sounds	Suspect pericardial effusion
Lungs	Persistent cough	Suspect pneumonia, especially in the infant
	Expiratory grunting	Suspect pneumonia
	Subcostal or intercostal retractions	Respiratory distress
	Flaring of nasal alae	Respiratory distress
Abdomen	Localized tenderness	Appendicitis, hepatitis, pyelonephritis
Extremities	Joint swelling, pain	Septic joint, arthritis
	Bone pain	Osteomyelitis, Leukemia, Sickle Cell Crisis
Integument	Petechial rashes, cellulitis	Meningococcemia, Rocky Mountain spotted fever, Leukemia

Gram Stain
Useful for classifying bacteria and thus narrowing the list of diagnostic possibilities. Organisms with recognizable structures such as some fungi and parasites can be identified without staining.

Cultures
Bacterial Fungi
Selective media is used to classify the bacteria or fungus as to type and subtype. This information can then be used to guide selection of a therapeutic agent.

Viral
Viral cultures are usually done in tissue cultures. This method can take significantly longer than that available for bacteria and fungi.

Immunologic Techniques
Immunofluorescence
Fluorescent antibodies (FA) are specific antisera that are used to identify some bacteria by the typical fluorescence that results when they are added to sera containing the suspected organism.

Agglutination Tests
A substance, usually latex, is coated with antibodies that will agglutinate when added to sera containing their antigen.

Countercurrent Immunoelectrophoresis (CCIE)
Is able to detect antigens in body fluids, including CSF and urine. It can identify antigens of *H influenzae* type b, *S pneumoniae*, and some types of *N meningitidis*. The latex agglutination is more sensitive and can also detect antigens of group B streptococcus.

ELISA
*e*nzyme-*l*inked *i*mmuno-*s*orbent *a*ssay is used to detect viral antibodies. It is now available for detecting most viruses. For HIV it is both sensitive and specific, but not absolutely certain, so confirmatory tests (eg Western blot) must be done.

Beta-lactamase production can be determined for staphylococci, *Hemophilus influenzae* and *Neisseria gonorrhoeae*. Its presence means a resistance to penicillin and ampicillin by the bacteria.

The Sepsis Work Up

A sepsis workup is done when a significant infection is feared and either an obvious source or the extent of the infection is not evident. It is a constellation of procedures selected to optimize identification of the cause and the extent of the infection, since these can influence selection of appropriate treatment. The components of the sepsis work up are:

Blood Cultures
A minimum of one blood culture is obtained.

Lumbar Puncture
CSF is sent for: Protein, Glucose, Culture and Sensitivity, CCIE, Cell Count, and other studies based on clinical suspicion

Chest X-ray
Obtained to rule out pneumonia, as well as other chest pathology. Not necessary in children when pneumonia is clinically ruled out, but critical in young infants.

Chem 7 (Na, K, Cl, CO$_2$, Glucose, BUN, Cr)
The glucose is needed for comparison with the CSF glucose, BUN and Cr to assess hydration status and guide dosing of potentially nephrotoxic drugs. Electrolytes provide guidance in fluid therapy and assess the potential of inappropriate ADH found in some cases of meningitis (especially *H influenzae*).

Urine
For Culture and Sensitivity as well as routine studies. It should be obtained by suprapubic tap in infants, or by bladder catheterization in children in whom a midstream clean catch urine cannot be obtained.

WBC
The white blood count can be supportive, but is not diagnostic of a bacterial infection. Typically the WBC is elevated in bacterial infections and normal or decreased in viral infections. However, early viral infections may have elevated WBCs and overwhelming bacterial infections may cause a decreased number of WBCs. Also other conditions such as leukemia can obscure the interpretation of the WBC. (CAUTION: an automated blood cell counter cannot differentiate between blast cells and lymphocytes and will report them as lymphocytes or monocytes.)

Pathophysiologic Manifestations

Febrile Patients at Increased Risk for Infectious Causes

Patient Group	At Risk For
Previously Normal	
Neonate < 1 month old	Group B streptococcus, *E coli, Listeria monocytogenes*, herpes simplex
Infant < 3 months old	Group B streptococcus, *E coli, Listeria monocytogenes*, respiratory syncytial virus, enterovirus, *H influenzae*, N meningitis
Temperature > 41 C	Meningitis, bacteremia, pneumonia, heat stroke, hemorrhagic shock-encephalopathy syndrome
Petechial rash with fever	Meningococcus, *Hemophilus influenzae* type b, pneumococcus, Rocky Mountain spotted fever
Immunocompromised	
Sickle cell anemia	Pneumococcal sepsis, meningitis, Salmonella
Asplenia	Encapsulated bacteria, esp. pneumococcus, Salmonella
Agammaglobulinemia	Bacteremia, sinopulmonary infection
AIDS	Pneumococcus, *H influenzae* type b, Salmonella
Immunosuppressive drugs	*Pseudomonas aeruginosa, S aureus, Candida, S epidermidis*
Left-to-right shunt heart lesions	endocarditis
Central venous lines	*S aureus, S epidermidis, Corynebacterium, Candida*

Summary of Selected Bacterial Infections by Age Groups

Infection	Most Common Pathogens	Initial Treatment
Sepsis/Meningitis		
< 2 months	group B streptococci *E coli* *Listeria monocytogenes* *N meningitidis* *S pneumoniae*	ampicillin and gentamicin OR ampicillin and cefotaxime
2 months - 8 years	*H influenzae* *N meningitidis* *S pneumoniae*	cefotaxime or ceftriaxone OR ampicillin and chloramphenicol
> 8 years	*N meningitidis* *S pneumoniae*	cefotaxime or ceftriaxone
Acute Otitis Media		
< 2 months	*S pneumoniae* *H influenzae* group A streptococci *S aureus* gram-negative enterics	ampicillin and gentamicin OR cefotaxime
> 2 months	*S pneumoniae* *H influenzae* *B catarrhalis* group A streptococci *S aureus*	amoxicillin OR erythromycin/ sulfisoxazole OR augmentin OR cefixime

Pneumonia

< 2 months	group B streptococci *S pneumoniae* *S aureus*	ampicillin and gentamicin OR ampicillin and cefotaxime
	Chlamydia trachomatis	erythromycin
2 months - 8 years	*S pneumoniae* *H influenzae* *S aureus* *Mycoplasma*	amoxicillin OR erythromycin/ sulfisoxazole OR cefaclor OR cefixime OR augmentin
> 8 years	*S pneumoniae* *Mycoplasma*	erythromycin

Urinary Tract Infection

| < 2 months | Assume neonatal sepsis until proved otherwise and treat as above. | |
| > 2 months | *E coli*
Proteus species
Klebsiella species
Staphylococcus epidermidis
Enterococci | amoxicillin OR trimethoprim/
sulfamethaxazole OR
cephalexin OR sulfisoxazole
OR nitrofurantoin |

Osteomyelitis

| All Ages | *S aureus*
S pneumoniae
H influenzae | begin antibiotic to cover
S aureus (oxacillin or
nafcillin); switch antibiotic
as indicated by culture and
sensitivities |

Septic Arthritis

< 2 months	*S aureus* group B streptococcus gram-negative enterics	nafcillin/oxacillin and gentamicin
2 months - 8 years	*H influenzae* *S aureus* Streptococcal species	nafcillin/oxacillin and ceftriaxone
> 8 years	*S aureus* *Neisseria gonorrhoeae*	nafcillin/oxacillin and ceftriaxone

Special Groups

< 5 years	*H influenzae*	base on culture and sensitivity
sickle cell	salmonella	
puncture wound of foot	*Pseudomonas aeruginosa*	

CHAPTER 8

Childhood Exanthems

Disease	Incubation Period	Typical Distribution	Clinical Features
Maculopapular lesions			
•Measles (Rubeola)	10 - 14 days	Begins at hairline and descends downward; Generalized by 3rd day; Confluent on face, neck, upper trunk	3 day prodrome with 3 C's: Cough, Conjunctivitis, Coryza; Koplik's spots 2 days before rash; desquamates after 7-10 days
•Rubella (German measles, 3 day measles)	14 - 21 days	Begins on face, progresses rapidly downward; Generalized by second day; Fades in order of appearance	Postauricular, suboccipital lymphadenopathy; Arthritis common in women
•Roseola (exanthema subitum)	10 - 14 days	Appears after defervescence of fever; initially on chest, then face, extremities; fades rapidly	3-4 day prodrome of high fever in otherwise well appearing 1 to 4 year old child
•Erythema infectiosum (Fifth disease; caused by parvovirus B19)	7 - 14 days	Red flushed cheeks with circumoral pallor (slapped cheek); followed by reticular, lacy rash on extremities; may recur on exposure to trauma, sunlight, heat	Patients with diseases that shorten RBC life span may have an aplastic crisis
•Enterovirus (especially Echovirus type 9)	few days	Rubella-like lesions; nonpuritic; may be petechial; lasts 3-5 days	Fever, malaise, sore throat, rhinorrhea, vomiting, diarrhea, herpangina; illness may mimic meningococcemia
•Scarlet fever (Group A streptococci)	2 - 4 days	Sandpaper texture; appears 1st on flexor surfaces, then generalized; most intense on neck, shoulders, axilla, inguinal, popliteal skin folds, circumoral pallor, lasts 7 days then desquamates	Pharyngitis, tonsillitis, strawberry tongue, palatal petechiae
Vesicular/pustular lesions			
•Varicella (Chickenpox)	14 - 21 days	Discrete puritic macules which progress to vesicles, umbilicated pustules and then crusted lesions; all stages are present at the same time; can involve mucous membranes	Avoid aspirin. Contagious until all lesions are crusted over.
•*Herpes zoster* (shingles)		Erythema followed by red papules, then vesicles in 12-24 hours, then pustules in 72 hours, then crusts in 10-12 days; unilateral peripheral dermatome distribution; does not cross midline	History of varicella Pre-eruptive pain common
•Hand, foot and mouth syndrome (*Coxsackievirus* A16)	4 - 6 days	Palmar and plantar pustules have typical elliptical football-shaped appearance	Fever, myalgia, malaise, herpangina, rhinorrhea, vomiting, diarrhea
•Disseminated gonococcemia		Erythematous or hemorrhagic papules that evolve into pustules or vesicles with an erythematous halo	Affects primarily young women; Fever and migratory polyarthralgias are common
•Impetigo (group A streptococcus; bullous lesions are caused by *Staphylococci*)		Honey-colored crusted lesions with predilection for face and exposed areas; bullous lesions are round bullae which rupture quickly	Poststreptococcal glomerulonephritis is potential complication; Bullous impetigo may be mistaken for cigarette burns
•Insect bites		Local reactions may resemble infectious exanthems or may be secondarily infected	

118

Disease Profiles

Systemic Infections

Occult Bacteremia
Presence of bacteria in the bloodstream without clinical manifestations other than fever.
> **Etiology**
>> *S pneumoniae* (70-80%), *H influenzae* type b, *N meningitidis*, Group A streptococcus, *S aureus*
> **Predisposing Conditions**
>> Age 3 months to 2 years
>> Only 4% in this age group with fever have occult bacteremia.
> **Symptoms**
>> Fever (usually > 102 F), irritability, no localizing signs
> **Laboratory Findings**
>> WBC < 5,000 or > 15,000, low colony count positive blood culture
> **Diagnostic Plan**
>> Blood culture, CBC
> **Therapeutic Plan**
>> If organism not *S pneumoniae*, treat as sepsis: complete sepsis workup if not done and begin antibiotics appropriate for age.
>> If organism is *S pneumoniae* and child is afebrile when culture results become known, repeat culture and begin PO antibiotics. If child still febrile, complete sepsis workup, repeat blood culture and decide on in-patient or out-patient treatment based on age and condition of child.
> **Prognosis**
>> Spontaneous resolution in 24 to 48 hours with *S pneumoniae*; sepsis with other organisms.

Sepsis
Life-threatening invasion of the bloodstream which may seed local areas.
> **Etiology**
>> *H influenzae* and *N meningitidis*, and *S pneumoniae* are most common
> **Predisposing Conditions**
>> compromised host defense, immaturity
> **Symptoms**
>> high fever, local pain (if invasive)
> **Physical Findings**
>> petechial rash

Laboratory Findings
>   WBC > 15,000 with shift to left, positive blood culture

Potential Complications
>   meningitis, osteomyelitis, septic joint

Diagnostic Plan
>   sepsis work up

Therapeutic Plan
>   Antibiotic choice is age specific; see table - Childhood Exanthems in this chapter

Central Nervous System Infections

Meningitis
Inflammation of the meninges

Etiology
>   bacterial, aseptic, fungal, atypical bacterial

Pathophysiologic Abnormality
>   inflammation of the meninges

Symptoms
>   severe headache, altered sensorium, seizures, vomiting

Physical Findings
>   meningeal signs (nuchal rigidity, Kernig's or Brudzinski's signs) bulging fontanelle, seizures

Bacterial Meningitis

Etiology
>   age specific: see table - Childhood Exanthems in this chapter

Pathophysiologic Abnormality
>   usually hematogenously seeded

Laboratory Findings
>   Elevated CSF WBCs, elevated CSF protein, decreased CSF glucose, positive CSF culture and Gram stain, positive latex agglutination test, positive CCIE

Potential Complications
>   shock, DIC, subdural effusion, cerebral edema, seizures, SIADH, neurologic sequelae

Diagnostic Plan
>   sepsis work up

Therapeutic Plan
>   Antibiotic choice is age specific; see table - Childhood Exanthems in this chapter

Aseptic Meningitis
Non bacterial inflammation of the meninges
>   **Etiology**
>   >   Viruses
>   >   >   Enteroviruses (85% of cases)
>   >   >   >   coxsackie virus
>   >   >   >   echoviruses
>   >   >   Arboviruses
>   >   >   >   St. Louis encephalitis virus
>   >   >   >   California encephalitis virus
>   >   >   HIV
>   >   >   Varicella
>   >   >   Epstein-Barr virus
>   >   >   lymphocytic choriomeningitis
>   >   >   measles
>   >   >   rubella
>   >   >   rabies
>   >   >   influenza
>   >   >   parainfluenza
>   >   >   CMV
>   >   >   mumps
>   >   *Mycoplasma*
>   >   *Chlamydia*
>   >   Various fungi, protozoa and other parasites
>   >   postinfectious reactions to various viruses
>   >   Less common causes include: leptospirosis, syphilis, Lyme disease, Cat-scratch fever, nocardiosis, Rocky Mountain spotted fever, vasculitis, intracranial hemorrhage, reactions to NSAIDS and heavy metal poisoning

>   **Symptoms**
>   >   headache, irritability, fever, nausea, vomiting, retrobulbar pain

>   **Physical Findings**
>   >   nuchal rigidity, exanthems, signs of underlying disease

>   **Laboratory Findings**
>   >   elevated CSF WBCs (often predominately polymorphonuclear cells early, lymphocytes and mononuclear cells later), Normal or slightly elevated CSF protein, normal CSF glucose in viral causes, negative CSF Gram stain

>   **Therapeutic Plan**
>   >   supportive, if viral cause

>   **Prognosis**
>   >   usually self limiting if viral cause

Encephalitis
An acute inflammation of brain parenchyma
> **Etiology**
>> *Herpes simplex*, St. Louis encephalitis virus, California encephalitis virus, eastern equine encephalitis virus, western equine encephalitis virus, coxsackie virus, echoviruses; postinfectious encephalitis following measles, mumps, Varicella, rubella; *Mycoplasma pneumoniae, Toxoplasma gondii*
> **Symptoms**
>> similar to aseptic meningitis, but more severe CNS manifestations: confusion, delirium, hallucinations, memory loss, combativeness, seizures and coma
> **Physical Findings**
>> focal neurologic signs: ataxia, signs of increased intracranial pressure
> **Laboratory Findings**
>> increased CSF RBCs with *Herpes simplex*; increased CSF WBCs (usually 10 - 500), increased CSF protein, normal CSF glucose
> **Diagnostic Plan**
>> Brain biopsy may be indicated if *Herpes simplex* is suspected
> **Therapeutic Plan**
>> Acyclovir for *Herpes simplex* and complicated *herpes zoster*; other etiologies generally supportive care for increased ICP
> **Prognosis**
>> St. Louis, California, western equine encephalitis: good
>> Eastern equine, *Herpes simplex* encephalitis: 60% death, high incidence of serious neurologic sequelae

Facial Infections

Causes of Acute Periorbital Swelling

Infections	Noninfectious
Sty/chalazion	Trauma
Conjunctivitis	Allergy
Dacrocystitis/dacroadenitis	Insect bite
Periorbital/orbital cellulitis	

Periorbital Cellulitis
inflammatory process occurring in the structures superficial to the orbital septum

Etiology
bacterial pathogen identified in only 30% of cases: three common routes of infection -- infecting organism may be related to each route
- trauma or insect bite -- *S aureus* or *Streptococcus pyogenes*
- extension from a sinusitis -- *H influenzae* or *S pneumoniae*
- bactermia with seeding of tissues -- *H influenzae* or *S pneumoniae*

Symptoms
no pain with movement of eyes

Physical Findings
inflammation of eyelids and periorbital tissues; no proptosis

Potential Complications
orbital cellulitis

Differential Diagnosis
trauma, periorbital edema, local allergic reactions

Therapeutic Plan
oral antibiotics to cover likely etiologic agents; careful monitoring to detect progression to orbital cellulitis

Prognosis
good if non progressive

Orbital Cellulitis
Inflammatory process deep to the orbital septum

Etiology
H influenzae, Streptococcus, Pneumococcus, *S aureus*

Symptoms
pain with movement of eyes, fever

Physical Findings
inflammation of eyelids and periorbital tissues; proptosis; chemosis

Laboratory Findings
leukocytosis

Potential Complications
cavernous sinus thrombosis; meningitis; epidural, subdural or brain abscess

Diagnostic Plan
sepsis work up

Therapeutic Plan
IV antibiotics, ophthalmologic consult

Buccal Cellulitis
Except for the location, the implications of this entity parallel those of periorbital cellulitis

___

Oral Infections

Candidal Gingivostomatitis
>   **Alternate Terminology**
>>   thrush
>   **Etiology**
>>   Candida species, usually *Candida albicans*
>   **Predisposing Conditions**
>>   common in infants, if occurs after infancy, consider immune deficiency
>   **Symptoms**
>>   decreased feeding in infants
>   **Physical Findings**
>>   grayish-white lesions on buccal mucosa and dorsum of tongue
>   **Laboratory Findings**
>>   pseudohyphae on Gram stain, *Candida* on culture
>   **Therapeutic Plan**
>>   nystatin oral suspension

Herpetic Gingivostomatitis
>   **Alternate Terminology**
>>   cold sores
>   **Etiology**
>>   *Herpes simplex*; usually type I, may be type II
>   **Pathogenesis**
>>   primary infection involves the mouth and gums, recurrent infections the lips
>   **Pathophysiologic Abnormality**
>>   after primary infection the virus lies dormant in nerve tissue until reactivated
>   **Predisposing Conditions**
>>   recurrence is precipitated by stress, either physical or emotional
>   **Symptoms**
>>   fever to 105 F, painful lesions
>   **Physical Findings**
>>   erythematous, edematous, ulcerative lesions in mouth
>   **Chronologic Sequence of Manifestations**
>>   Incubation period 3-9 days; improves after 3-10 days; resolves in 2 weeks
>   **Potential Complications**
>>   dehydration

Therapeutic Plan

cold foods and liquids, mixture of Maalox and Benadryl, analgesics, IV fluids sometimes needed

Herpangina

Alternate Terminology

Hand, foot, mouth when characteristic lesions are also on those locations

Etiology

Coxsackie virus types A & B; echoviruses

Symptoms

headache, myalgia, fever, sore throat, dysphagia, vomiting

Physical Findings

temperature to 106 F, ulcerative lesions on posterior pharynx, tonsilar pillars and soft palate

Chronologic Sequence of Manifestations

fever lasts 3-5 days, lesions may last a week

Potential Complications

dehydration

Therapeutic Plan

symptomatic, cool foods and liquids, analgesics

Necrotizing Ulcerative Gingivitis

Alternate Terminology

Vincent's stomatitis, trench mouth

Etiology

fusiform bacilli and spirochetes invading areas of interdental papillae eroded by plaque

Predisposing Conditions

severe dental plaque

Physical Findings

fever, malodorous breath, gingival pain

Therapeutic Plan

penicillin G

Upper Respiratory Infections

Sinusitis

Etiology

S pneumoniae, unencapsulated strains of *H influenzae, B catarrhalis*

Pathophysiologic Abnormality
> frontal sinuses are not developed until school age; maxillary sinusitis rare before 18 months

Predisposing Conditions
> allergic rhinitis, URI, swimming, trauma

Symptoms
> fever, headache, chronic rhinorrhea, malodorous nasal discharge, persistent cough

Physical Findings
> purulent rhinorrhea, periorbital swelling, localized tenderness, malodorous breath

Laboratory Findings
> sinus X-ray: air fluid levels, opacity of sinus

Potential Complications
> orbital cellulitis, meningitis, brain abscess, cavernous sinus thrombosis

Therapeutic Plan
> amoxicillin, trimethoprim/sulfamethoxazole

Acute Otitis Media

Alternate Terminology
> suppurative otitis media if membrane is perforated

Etiology
> *S pneumoniae*, unencapsulated *H influenzae*, *B catarrhalis*, Group A streptococcus, *S aureus*

Predisposing Conditions
> eustachian tube dysfunction leading to adsorption of air from middle ear leaving a vacuum

Symptoms
> URI symptoms, ear pain, fever, hearing impairment, vomiting, diarrhea

Physical Findings
> erythematous, bulging, non mobile TM

Potential Complications
> hearing deficit with impaired language acquisition

Therapeutic Plan
> amoxicillin

Streptococcal Pharyngitis

Etiology
> group A beta hemolytic streptococcus

Symptoms
> fever, sore throat, headache, abdominal pain

Physical Findings

fever, exudative tonsillar hypertrophy, petechiae on soft palate, tender anterior cervical nodes

Laboratory Findings

positive rapid strep screen, positive culture

Potential Complications

otitis media, acute sinusitis, peritonsillar abscess, cervical lymphadenitis, acute rheumatic fever, acute glomerulonephritis

Differential Diagnosis

viral pharyngitis, *Corynebacterium diphtheriae*, *M pneumoniae*, Infectious mononucleosis, *N gonorrhoeae* opportunistic infections in leukemia

Diagnostic Plan

rapid strep screen, throat culture

Therapeutic Plan

penicillin po for 10 days

Viral Pharyngitis

Etiology

Epstein-Barr virus, adenovirus, *Herpes simplex* virus, enterovirus, influenza virus, parainfluenza virus, measles

Symptoms

indistinguishable from strep. pharyngitis

Physical Findings

indistinguishable from strep. pharyngitis

Therapeutic Plan

symptomatic

Infectious Mononucleosis

Etiology

Epstein-Barr virus

Symptoms

malaise, headache, fever, sore throat, fatigue, abdominal pain

Physical Findings

pharyngitis, tender anterior and posterior cervical nodes, splenomegaly, maculopapular rash

Laboratory Findings

positive monospot test, antibodies to EBV (titers more sensitive in patients < 5 years)

Potential Complications
>   splenic rupture, hepatitis, airway obstruction, aseptic meningitis, Guillain-Barré syndrome

Therapeutic Plan
>   avoid contact sports until spleen normal

Acute Epiglottitis

Etiology
>   *H influenzae* type b

Pathophysiologic Abnormality
>   infectious edema of the epiglottis

Predisposing Conditions
>   age 2-7 years, lack of Hib vaccine

Symptoms
>   rapid onset: fever, sore throat

Physical Findings
>   respiratory distress, stridor, drooling, sitting forward with mouth open, cherry red epiglottis (should only be viewed in Operating Room)

Laboratory Findings
>   lateral soft tissue neck X-ray: characteristic Thumb sign

Chronologic Sequence of Manifestations
>   symptoms and findings evolve in hours from none to life threatening

Potential Complications
>   complete airway obstruction

Differential Diagnosis
>   visualization under controlled conditions should not be delayed by diagnostic tests

Diagnostic Plan
>   transport to an Operating Room where anesthesiology and ENT personnel are available; avoid agitation

Therapeutic Plan
>   Endotracheal intubation; ventilatory support; IV antibiotics to cover beta-lactamase producing organisms

Prognosis
>   good if airway controlled and antibiotics effective

Acute Laryngotracheobronchitis

Alternate Terminology
>   viral croup

Etiology

respiratory viruses; parainfluenza most common

Pathophysiologic Abnormality

laryngeal edema

Symptoms

hoarseness, barking cough, fever, URI symptoms

Physical Findings

inspiratory stridor, respiratory distress

Laboratory Findings

Lateral neck soft tissue X-ray: subglottic narrowing (penciling)

Chronologic Sequence of Manifestations

symptoms progress over days; often worse at night

Therapeutic Plan

humidified air; racemic epinephrine if hospitalized; corticosteriods

Lower Respiratory Infections

Bronchiolitis

Etiology

respiratory syncytial virus (50%); parainfluenza virus; adenovirus

Pathophysiologic Abnormality

infectious edema of bronchiolar mucosa; bronchospasm is not a component

Predisposing Conditions

rare after 2 years age

Symptoms

cough, wheezing, dyspnea, feeding difficulty

Physical Findings

wheezing, flaring of nasal alae, crackles; may have cyanosis

Laboratory Findings

rapid viral antigen assays

Chronologic Sequence of Manifestations

mild URI symptoms followed by progression of respiratory distress

Potential Complications

apnea, respiratory failure

Differential Diagnosis

Asthma (rare under 9 months), foreign body aspiration, pertussis, CHF, pneumonia

Diagnostic Plan

pulse oximeter, chest X-ray

Therapeutic Plan

O_2 and IV fluids if needed

Ribavirin, bronchodilators and steroids may all be considered

Prognosis
>   may be prone to asthma later in life

Pneumonia
>   **Etiology**
>   >   Bacterial, viral, fungal, rickettsiae agents
>   **Pathophysiologic Abnormality**
>   >   infection of lung parenchyma

Bacterial Pneumonia
>   **Etiology**
>   >   *S pneumoniae, H influenzae* type b, Group A streptococcus
>   **Symptoms**
>   >   abrupt fever, shaking chills, cough, chest pain
>   **Physical Findings**
>   >   crackles, decreased breath sounds, flaring of nasal alae, grunting respirations
>   **Laboratory Findings**
>   >   consolidation on chest X-ray; leukocytosis; blood cultures may be positive
>   **Therapeutic Plan**
>   >   age specific; see table above

Viral Pneumonia
>   **Etiology**
>   >   RSV most common; other respiratory viruses
>   **Therapeutic Plan**
>   >   Ribavirin for severe RSV pneumonia
>   >   Acyclovir for severe herpesvirus pneumonia
>   >   Amantidine for influenza pneumonia

Mycoplasma Pneumonia
>   **Etiology**
>   >   *M pneumoniae*
>   **Predisposing Conditions**
>   >   peak age: 5-15 years
>   **Symptoms**
>   >   sore throat, non productive cough, fever, headache, malaise
>   **Physical Findings**
>   >   may have few signs

Laboratory Findings
> cold agglutinins positive; chest X-ray: interstitial infiltrate

Therapeutic Plan
> erythromycin

P Carinii Pneumonia

Etiology
> *P carinii*

Predisposing Conditions
> immune compromised patient

Symptoms
> exertional dyspnea is characteristic in older patients; severe respiratory distress with cyanosis in infants

Laboratory Findings
> tracheal washings positive

Therapeutic Plan
> trimethoprim-sulfamethoxazole

Cardiac Infections

Endocarditis

Etiology
> Alpha-hemolytic streptococcus, *S aureus*, *S epidermidis*

Predisposing Conditions
> central venous lines, injecting drug use, valvular heart lesions, cardiac shunts with high turbulence

Symptoms
> fatigue, fever, malaise

Physical Findings
> Roth's spots, Janeway lesions and Osler's nodes are rare; changing murmurs, splinter hemorrhages

Laboratory Findings
> positive blood cultures; vegetations seen on echocardiogram

Potential Complications
> emboli, mycotic aneurysms, CHF

Therapeutic Plan
> long-term IV antibiotics (at least 4 weeks)

Myocarditis

Etiology

enteroviruses (coxsackie B, echovirus)

Symptoms

fever, symptoms of CHF

Physical Findings

dysrhythmias, signs of CHF, abnormal EKG

Laboratory Findings

EKG: ST segment depression, T-wave inversion; Chest X-ray: cardiomegaly, pulmonary vascular congestion, edema

Potential Complications

Coxsackie myocarditis is extremely sensitive to digitalis; regular digitalizing doses can be highly toxic

Therapeutic Plan

supportive treatment

Prognosis

spontaneous resolution in 10-20%. 50% of untreated older patients die within 2 years; 80% die within 8 years.

Pericarditis

Etiology

Bacteria, viruses, fungi and tuberculosis

Pathophysiologic Abnormality

inflammation with fluid accumulation in the pericardial sac

Symptoms

left shoulder pain, back pain, relieved by sitting forward, fever, cough, dyspnea

Physical Findings

pericardial friction rub, distant heart sounds

Laboratory Findings

echo: pericardial fluid; chest X-ray: enlarged heart with normal pulmonary vascularity; EKG: ST segment elevation

Potential Complications

cardiac tamponade

Therapeutic Plan

pericardial drainage, antibiotics if bacterial etiology

Gastrointestinal System Infections

Hepatitis A
    Alternate Terminology
        infectious hepatitis
    Etiology
        HAV; an RNA virus
    Symptoms
        may be mistaken for a cold in children; fever, RUQ pain, anorexia, nausea, vomiting, diarrhea
    Physical Findings
        Jaundice, hepatomegaly, RUQ tenderness
    Laboratory Findings
        elevated liver transaminases, elevated direct and indirect bilirubin, positive hepatitis A-IgM indicates acute disease
    Chronologic Sequence of Manifestations
        incubation period: 2-6 weeks; prodromal phase may not be noticed in children; GI symptoms, dark urine, jaundice subsides after 1-2 weeks
    Potential Complications
        fulminant hepatitis
    Differential Diagnosis
        infectious mononucleosis, leptospirosis, CMV, Wilson's disease, other viral hepatitis
    Therapeutic Plan
        supportive measures; enteric isolation
    Prognosis
        generally good in children
    Prevention
        exposed household contacts should get IgG within 2 weeks of contact; also a HAV vaccine became available in February 1995

Hepatitis B
    Alternate Terminology
        serum hepatitis
    Etiology
        HBV; DNA virus
    Symptoms
        fever, arthralgia, RUQ pain, anorexia, nausea, vomiting, diarrhea
    Physical Findings
        Jaundice, hepatomegaly, RUQ tenderness

Laboratory Findings
> elevated liver transaminases, elevated direct and indirect bilirubin, positive hepatitis B surface antigen (HB_sAg) indicates acute disease; antibodies against the hepatitis B surface antigen (HB_sAb) indicates immunity; presence of HB_eAg indicated infectivity

Chronologic Sequence of Manifestations
> incubation period: 2-6 months; GI symptoms, dark urine, jaundice subsides after 1-2 weeks

Potential Complications
> fulminant hepatitis, carrier state, chronic active hepatitis (predisposes to hepatocellular carcinoma)

Differential Diagnosis
> infectious mononucleosis, leptospirosis, CMV, Wilson's disease, other viral hepatitis

Therapeutic Plan
> supportive measures; enteric isolation

Prognosis
> generally good in children

Prevention
> HBV vaccine

Urinary Tract Infections

Cystitis

Etiology
> *E coli*, other intestinal organisms

Predisposing Conditions
> female, anatomic abnormalities

Symptoms
> dysuria, urgency, frequency

Laboratory Findings
> positive urine culture

Potential Complications
> pyelonephritis

Therapeutic Plan
> oral antibiotics

Pyelonephritis
    Symptoms
        gastrointestinal symptoms common, fever, chills, flank pain
    Physical Findings
        CVA tenderness
    Potential Complications
        hypertension, renal insufficiency if severe renal damage
    Therapeutic Plan
        IV antibiotics if toxic

Joint Infections

Septic Arthritis
    Alternate Terminology
        septic arthritis
    Etiology
        S aureus: often preceded by trauma
        H influenzae: most common in children < 5 years; often associated with infection elsewhere, eg, meningitis, otitis media
        Streptococci: group A, B, anaerobic, *Streptococcus viridans*
        *S p*neumoniae, *N gonorrhoeae*: primarily hands, wrist, knee, ankle
        gram-negative enteric: neonates, immunosuppressed
        Pseudomonas organisms: immunosuppressed, neonates, puncture wounds
    Pathophysiologic Abnormality
        bacterial invasion of joint space
    Symptoms
        fever, irritability, joint pain, may appear toxic
    Physical Findings
        joint effusion, swelling, limitation of motion
    Laboratory Findings
        ESR elevated, blood cultures positive (50% of time), WBC may be elevated
        Joint aspirate: WBC > 50,000, Glucose < 50% of blood glucose; poor mucin clot
        X-ray: bone demineralization (late finding) joint distension
        Bone scan: Technetium: positive within 24 hours may be able to differentiate osteomyelitis
        Gallium: positive within 24-48 hours; becomes normal with effective treatment
    Potential Complications
        destruction of cartilage, growth plate
    Differential Diagnosis
        see chapter on musculoskeletal disorders

Therapeutic Plan
    see table - Summary of Selected Bacterial Infections by Age Groups in this
        chapter for antibiotic choices
    Surgical drainage often required
Prognosis
    better the sooner effective treatment is begun

Bone Infections

Osteomyelitis
Etiology
    similar to septic joint plus *Mycobacterium* and in immunocompromised patients,
    fungal
Pathophysiologic Abnormality
    predilection for metaphysis of long bones
Predisposing Conditions
    trauma, systemic bacterial infection, immunocompromised host, sickle cell
    disease, drug abuse
Symptoms
    fever, local pain; infants may have little systemic toxicity
Physical Findings
    local warmth, swelling, tenderness; limp; restricted movement
Laboratory Findings
    WBC may be elevated; ESR elevated; blood culture positive > 50% of patients
    X-ray: soft tissue swelling in 3-4 days; bone changes in 7-10 days (periosteal
    elevation, lytic changes, sclerosis)
    Bone scan: technetium most helpful
Potential Complications
    chronic osteomyelitis; septic joint; growth plate damage
Differential Diagnosis
    septic arthritis, cellulitis, fracture, Ewing's tumor
Therapeutic Plan
    antibiotics determined by culture (initial coverage to include *S aureus*)

Disseminated Infections

Rocky Mountain Spotted Fever
Etiology
    Rickettsia rickettsii

Pathophysiologic Abnormality
> diffuse vasculitis

Predisposing Conditions
> tick bite

Symptoms
> fever, chills, headache, irritability, confusion, delirium, myalgia, photophobia

Physical Findings
> conjunctivitis, profuse nonpitting edema, rash: rose-colored maculas beginning on wrists, hands, ankles and feet (involves palms and soles), then becoming petechial and purpuric over entire body

Laboratory Findings
> hyponatremia, thrombocytopenia, positive immunofluorescence antibody

Chronologic Sequence of Manifestations
> abrupt onset after 2- 8 day incubation period

Potential Complications
> neurologic deficits, coma, renal failure, DIC, gangrene of distal extremities, shock

Differential Diagnosis
> see meningococcemia

Therapeutic Plan
> tetracycline or chloramphenicol

Meningococcemia

Etiology
> *Neisseria meningitidis*

Symptoms
> fever, headache, malaise, arthralgia, vomiting

Physical Findings
> pink maculopapular rash; generalized petechiae, including palms and soles; (if purpura and ecchymosis expect high mortality)

Laboratory Findings
> scraping of purpuric lesion may have positive Gram stain and culture

Chronologic Sequence of Manifestations
> onset insidious to fulminant; may progress to death in 12 hours or less

Potential Complications
> meningitis; pericarditis, DIC, Waterhouse-Friderichsen syndrome, cardiovascular collapse, death

Differential Diagnosis

Rocky Mountain spotted fever, *H influenzae* (rarely), leukemia, idiopathic thrombocytopenic purpura, infectious mononucleosis, measles, Henoch-Schönlein purpura, viral infections

Therapeutic Plan

penicillin IV; respiratory isolation

Treatment of Contacts

rifampin

Acquired Immunodeficiency Syndrome

Discussed in Chapter 6

Peggy J Hines
A Eugene Osbum

Developmental Considerations

Infants are obligate nasal breathers. Complete occlusion of the nares can result in life-threatening apnea. Nasal obstruction can also interfere significantly with feeding in older infants since it is difficult to maintain an effective suck without patent nares.

In evaluating the symptoms of respiratory diseases in infants, remember to investigate the possibility of symptoms due to over-the-counter cold remedies. Sleep disturbances, irritability, etc. may be a side effect of the medication, not a manifestation of the condition.

Airway resistance to airflow is inversely proportional to the fourth power of the radius of the airway. Therefore, a given degree of tissue swelling causes more obstruction to air flow in the smaller child or infant.

The number of alveoli increases until age 10 to 12 years, but the number of bronchi do not increase after birth. Therefore, diseases which affect lung development can cause permanent ventilation perfusion mismatches if alveolar growth does not match that of the pulmonary vasculature development.

Males have smaller peripheral airways than females before school age, thus, pulmonary disease in male infants and children may be more severe than in females of the same age.

As soon as they can pick up objects, infants and toddlers are at risk for aspiration because they tend to put all small objects in their mouths.

Cardiac failure in infancy often presents as respiratory distress. Hepatomegaly in the infant with respiratory distress is the clue to congestive heart failure. Cardiac failure can be confirmed by cardiomegaly on chest X-ray.

Cyanosis due to congenital right-to-left shunts does not improve with 100% oxygen inhalation; that due to respiratory disorders generally does.

Upper airway obstruction is usually manifest by inspiratory stridor and increased inspiratory effort (retractions); obstruction below the glottis is usually manifest by expiratory stridor, and may be accompanied by prolonged expiration and wheezing. If the child is not hoarse, the obstruction is likely subglottic or tracheal.

Oxygen diffuses 20 times less readily across the capillary/alveolar surface than does carbon dioxide. Thus hypoxemia occurs relatively early in disorders of gas exchange and hypercapnia is a manifestation of a much more severe derangement of gas exchange.

Diagnostic Modalities
Blood Gas Analysis
Arterial Blood Gasses

PaO_2: values below 85 mm Hg breathing room air are abnormal, except in the very young infant. Respiratory failure is generally present when the value decreases to below 50 mm Hg.

$PaCO_2$: values above 45 mm Hg indicate hypoventilation, severe ventilation/perfusion mismatch or compensation for chronic metabolic acidosis.

O_2 saturation: Because of the nature of the oxyhemoglobin dissociation curve, oxygen saturation does not decrease appreciably until arterial PO_2 decreases to about 60 torr (mm Hg)

In obstructive airway disease, such as asthma, a deceptive phase occurs during progression through more severe obstruction. At the severe stage, the child may become quieter because of tiring and evolving CO_2 narcosis, the wheezing may diminish because not enough air is moved to make the noise, and the pH and PCO_2 are normal. The next phase, however, is respiratory failure as depicted in the figure below:

Progression of pH and Blood Gas Changes in Asthma			
Severity	**pH**	**PaO$_2$**	**PaCO$_2$**
Normal	7.40	98%	40 mm Hg
Mild	mildly elevated	normal	mild decrease
Moderate	elevated	decrease	decrease
Severe	normal	marked decrease	normal
Respiratory Failure	< 7.25	< 60 mm Hg	> 60 mm Hg

Alveolararterial PO$_2$ Difference:

The PAO_2 - PaO_2 difference is a measurement of gas exchange which is not influenced by minute volume. Increases in the difference is indicative of shunts between the pulmonary and systemic circulations.

Alveolar PO$_2$ (PAO_2) can be estimated by the formula:

$$PAO_2 = FiO_2 (P_B - 47) - PaO_2/R$$

where

FiO_2 = inspired percent of oxygen

P_B = barometric pressure

R = carbon dioxide production/oxygen consumption ratio: usually 0.8

Pulse Oximetry

A noninvasive method of monitoring O_2 saturation. However, it is affected by local vasoconstriction.

Radiography

Chest X-ray

A method for evaluation of structural aspects of the heart and lungs.

Lateral Neck Soft Tissue X-ray

Useful for evaluating causes of upper airway obstruction. Penciling of the trachea is common in croup. The "thumb sign" is suggestive of epiglottitis. Soft tissue changes may be seen in retropharyngeal abscesses.

Contrast Studies

Pulmonary arteriogram, bronchograms, thoracic aortograms, and barium swallows are sometimes useful in differentiating GI problems from pulmonary problems.

Radionuclide Lung Scans

These facilitate evaluation of pulmonary ventilation and perfusion.

Pulmonary Function Tests

In general, the child must be school age before he/she can cooperate sufficiently to perform these tests. When they can be done reliably, they are useful in identifying obstructive, restrictive or diffusion abnormalities. They are also helpful in quantitating response to bronchodilators. The more commonly used pulmonary function tests are:

Spirometer

Peak Expiratory Flow Rate (PEFR)

Forced Vital Capacity (FEV)

Forced Expiratory Volume in one second (FEV_1)

FEV_1/FEV ratio

Pneumography

One of the methods to assess neonatal apnea.

Flexible Bronchoscopy

Can be used with local anesthesia and thus in the ambulatory setting.

Rigid Bronchoscopy

Requires general sedation, but may be necessary for foreign body removal.

Lung Biopsy

May be required for histologic or culture diagnosis. Can be done with needle aspiration.

Sweat Chloride

Elevated in cystic fibrosis. False positive results are caused by adrenal insufficiency, malnutrition, ectodermal dysplasia, hypothyroidism, nephrogenic diabetes insipidus, mucopolysaccharidosis, Type I glycogen storage disease and fucosidosis.

Pathophysiologic Manifestations

Symptoms

Cough

A persistent cough is never normal in the neonate. A sudden onset of a paroxysmal cough should suggest foreign body aspiration.

Sputum Production

As a rule children swallow the mucus they produce and hence "do not produce" sputum.

Chest Pain

The pain may be a clue to the location of pathology, but be aware of referred pain in evaluating the patient.

Pleurisy

Pain associated with and exacerbated by inspiration. It may be difficult to differentiate from chest wall pain in children, and can be a cause of splinting with respiration.

Physical Findings

Respiratory Rate

Normal respiratory rates by age

Age	Breaths per Minute
Newborn	30-60
Infant 1-6 months	30-40
Infant 6-12 months	24-30
1-4 years	20-30
4-6 years	20-25
6-12 years	16-20
Over 12 years	12-16

Grunting

An expiratory grunt is a compensatory mechanism for loss of lung volume. It is never a normal finding. It may indicate pleural involvement and is seen sometimes with intraabdominal problems such as peritonitis.

Flaring of the Nasal Alae

This is a sign of increased airway resistance.

Subcostal Retractions

When small airway obstruction causes enough air trapping to depress the diaphragm, subcostal retractions will occur with inspiration.

Intercostal Retractions

This is a reflection of inspiration against increased lung compliance.

Tracheal Deviation

May reflect a pneumothorax or atelectasis. Can be a clue to foreign body aspiration.

Cervical Venous Distention

Seen in conditions causing persistent increased intrathoracic pressure and in cardiac tamponade.

Stridor

Is indicative of upper airway obstruction.

Thoracic Configuration

Chronic air trapping can produce a barrel chest configuration.

Breath Sounds

Normally the inspiration-to-expiration ratio is 2:1. This ratio is reversed in conditions resulting in bronchiolar obstruction.

Crackles/Rales

The term crackles is now preferred to rales. They are produced on inspiration by opening of small airways or alveoli.

Rhonchi/Wheezes

Expiratory noises which are prolonged rather than discrete sounds. Wheezes are higher pitched and may be musical in quality.

Clubbing of Nails

Most common pulmonary cause in children is cystic fibrosis.

Cyanosis

Cyanosis is the result of color changes due to the presence of at least 5 g of reduced Hb/dl. Central cyanosis is reflective of decreased oxygenation of the blood. It is due to a decreased oxygen saturation. Peripheral cyanosis is due to an increased arterial-venous oxygen difference and reflects local vascular stasis. The oxygen saturation is normal in peripheral cyanosis. Methemoglobin will produce cyanosis when it is exceeds more than 15% of the total hemoglobin.

Differential Considerations in Apnea of Infancy

SIDS

CNS Disorders

Seizures
Meningitis
Encephalitis
Intracranial hemorrhage (R/O shaken baby syndrome)
Increased intracranial pressure
Encephalopathy
Central hypoventilation

Pulmonary Disorders

Pneumonia (especially RSV, pertussis)
Pulmonary hemorrhage
Pulmonary edema

Cardiovascular Disorders

Dysrhythmias
Shock

Gastrointestinal Disorders

Gastroesophageal reflux
Tracheoesophageal fistula
Swallowing disorders

Metabolic Disorders

Hypoglycemia
Hypocalcemia
Hyponatremia
Inborn errors of metabolism

Musculoskeletal Disorders

Infant botulism
Guillain-Barré syndrome
Congenital myopathies

Other

Severe anemia
Poisoning
Hypothermia

Diagnostic Considerations in Respiratory Distress

UPPER AIRWAY DISEASE
    Congenital Causes
        Vascular ring
        Laryngeal web
        Vocal cord paralysis
        Laryngomalacia
        Tracheomalacia
        Micrognathia (Pierre Robin syndrome)
        Glossoptosis (Down syndrome, Beckwith- Wiedmann syndrome, hypothyroidism)
    Infectious Causes
        Croup
        Epiglottis
        Bacterial tracheitis
        Peritonsillar abscess
        Retropharyngeal abscess
        Diphtheria
    Traumatic Causes
        Foreign body
        Vocal cord paralysis
        Subglottic stenose
        Scald burns to pharynx, epiglottis
    Allergic Causes
        Angioneurotic edema
        Spasmodic croup

LOWER AIRWAY DISEASE
    Congenital Causes
        Cystic fibrosis
        Emphysema
        Diaphragmatic
    Infectious Causes
        Pneumonia
        Bronchiolitis
        Pleural effusions
        Empyema
    Allergic Causes
        Asthma
        Anaphylaxis
    Cardiovascular Causes
        Congestive heart failure
        Pulmonary edema
        Pulmonary embolism
        Polycythemia
        Severe anemia
    Traumatic Causes
        Bronchopulmonary dysplasia
        Foreign body
        Pneumothorax
        Pulmonary contusion
        Diaphragmatic defects
        Near drowning
        Spinal cord injury
    Neoplastic Causes
        Lung tumors
        Mediastinal masses
    Other Causes
        Sarcoidosis
        Musculoskeletal anomalies
        Scoliosis
        Pulmonary hemosiderosis

CENTRAL NERVOUS SYSTEM DISEASE
    Infectious Causes
        Meningitis
        Encephalitis
    Neuropathy/Myopathy Causes
        Guillain-Barré syndrome
        Werdnig-Hoffman syndrome
        Muscular dystrophy
        Myasthenia gravis
        Infant botulism
    Other Causes
        Seizures
        Poisonings

METABOLIC DISEASE
    Metabolic Acidosis
        Inborn errors of metabolism
        Diabetes mellitus
        Sepsis
        Dehydration
        Salicylism
        Other toxins
    Increased Oxygen Demand
        fever
        hyperthyroidism

Mediastinal Masses

Superior Mediastinum

Cystic hygroma
Vascular tumors
Neurogenic tumors
Thymic tumors
Teratomas
Hemangioma
Mediastinal abscess
Aortic aneurysm
Intrathoracic thyroid
Esophageal lesion

Anterior Mediastinum

Thymoma
Thymic hyperplasia
Thymic cyst
Teratoma
Lymphoma
Vascular tumor
Intrathoracic thyroid
Pleuropericardial cyst
Lymphadenopathy

Posterior Mediastinum

Neurogenic tumors
Enterogenous cysts
Thoracic
    meningocele
Aortic aneurysm

Middle Mediastinum

Lymphoma
Hypertrophic lymph nodes
Granuloma
Bronchogenic cyst
Enterogenic cysts
Metastasis
Pericardial cyst
Aortic aneurysm
Anomalies of great vessels

Recurrent or Persistent Respiratory Symptoms in Children

Indicators of Serious Chronic Respiratory Disease

Persistent fever
Limiting activity
Growth failure
Inadequate weight gain
Clubbing of digits
Persistent purulent sputum production
Sustained hypoxemia
Persistent infiltrates on X-ray
Persistent abnormalities in PFTs

Cough: Recurrent or Persistent

Differential Diagnosis

Recurrent Cough

Asthma
Drainage from upper airways
Aspiration
Frequent recurrent respiratory infections

Persistent Cough

Postinfection hypersensitivity
Asthma
Chronic sinusitis
Bronchiectasis
Foreign body aspiration
Gastroesophageal reflux
Pertussis
Tracheoesophageal fistula
Extrinsic compression of tracheobronchial tract
Habit cough
Tracheomalacia
Tuberculosis

CHAPTER 9

Wheezing: Recurrent or Persistent

Differential Diagnosis

Asthma

Other Hypersensitivity Reactions:

> Hypersensitivity pneumonitis
> Tropical eosinophilia
> Visceral larva migrans
> Allergic aspergillosis

Aspiration

> Foreign body
> Food, saliva, gastric contents
> Laryngotracheoesophageal cleft
> Tracheoesophageal fistula, H-type
> Neuromuscular weakness

Cystic Fibrosis

Cardiac Failure

Bronchiolitis Obliterans

Extrinsic Compression of Airways

> Vascular ring
> Enlarged lymph node
> Mediastinal tumor
> Lung cyst

Cigarette Smoke

Gastroesophageal Reflux

Sequelae of Bronchopulmonary Dysplasia

Tracheobronchomalacia

Stridor: Recurrent or Persistent

Differential Diagnosis

Recurrent   **Persistent**

Spasmodic Croup   Laryngeal Obstruction
                                              Laryngomalacia
Respiratory Infections   Papillomas
                                              Cysts
Laryngomalacia   Laryngeal webs
                                              Bilateral abductor paralysis of cords
                                              Foreign body

                                       Tracheobronchial Disease

                                              Tracheomalacia
                                              Subglottic tracheal webs
                                              Endotracheal tumors
                                              Subglottic tracheal stenosis
                                              Extrinsic masses

                                       Tracheoesophageal Fistula

                                       Other

                                              Gastroesophageal reflux
                                              Pierre Robin syndrome
                                              Cri du chat syndrome
                                              Hysterical stridor

Disease Profiles

Laryngomalacia
    Alternate Terminology
        infantile larynx, congenital laryngeal stridor
    Etiology
- congenital anomaly
- most common congenital laryngeal abnormality

    Pathophysiologic Abnormality
        abnormally small &/or soft larynx
    Symptoms
- stridor, noisy crowing respirations
- symptoms worse with URIs

    Laboratory Findings
        diagnosed by direct laryngoscopy
    Potential Complications
        difficulty feeding; rare need for tracheostomy
    Differential Diagnosis
        malformations of laryngeal cartilages, intraluminal webs, neck and chest neoplasms, vascular rings, cysts
    Therapeutic Plan
        reassurance of parents; slow careful feedings if needed
    Prognosis
        good; stridor usually resolved by 18 months of age

Bronchopulmonary Dysplasia
    Alternate Terminology
        BPD
    Etiology
- barotrauma: prolonged mechanical ventilation
- oxygen toxicity (requiring $FiO_2 > 0.8$)
- other predisposing conditions:
    * hyaline membrane disease
    * lower gestational age
    * male sex
    * patent ductus arteriosus
    * pulmonary infection (*Ureaplasma urealyticum*)
    * pulmonary edema

Pathophysiologic Abnormality

airway smooth muscle hypertrophy; interstitial edema from endothelial injury

Predisposing Conditions

oxygen and mechanical ventilations treatment of hyaline membrane disease

Physical Findings

tachypnea, wheezing, crackles, retractions, cyanosis

Laboratory Findings

- chest X-ray: characteristic fibrotic and cystic interstitial changes in the chronic stage
- ABGs: hypoxemia on room air

Potential Complications

cor pulmonale, pulmonary hypertension, growth retardation

Therapeutic Plan

oxygen to maintain PaO_2 in 60-80 mm Hg range, diuretics, bronchodilators, calorie supplementation, influenza and pneumococcal vaccine at appropriate ages

Prognosis

may require oxygen supplementation for a year after hospital discharge; may acquire normal pulmonary function by school age; prone to asthma

Cystic Fibrosis

Alternate Terminology

mucoviscidosis

Etiology

- autosomal recessive defect
- mutation of both alleles of CF gene (on chromosome 7)
- resultant abnormality in gene product:
cystic fibrosis membrane conductor (CFTR)
- 70% of mutations in North Americans is a three base pair deletion resulting in the absence of phenylalanine at codon 508 (Δ F 508)

Pathophysiologic Abnormality

abnormal control of chloride channels in epithelial cells of the pancreas, sweat and salivary glands, intestine, and reproductive and respiratory tracts.

- hypothesized that the function of the chloride channel determines the hydration of the mucous gel; inadequate hydration of the cell surface believed to result in inspissated secretions and organ damage in the pancreas, biliary tree, and lungs.

Epidemiology
- abnormalities of CF gene occurs in 1 of 25 people of Northern European extraction
- heterozygote carriers are asymptomatic
- CF occurs in 1 in 2500 live births
- frequency less in other populations, rare in African and Asian populations

Presenting Symptoms

failure to thrive (malabsorption); recurrent respiratory disease, cough, clubbing; meconium ileus (5-10%); obstructive jaundice; hyponatremia dehydration; rectal prolapse (20%); family history (sibling with CF; nasal polyps (10%)

Laboratory Findings
- sweat chloride > 60 mEq/L
- genetic testing using polymerase chain reaction (PCR) can detect 90% of abnormal genotypes reliably

Potential Complications

meconium ileus, intestinal obstruction, malnutrition, diabetes mellitus (8-12%); recurrent respiratory tract infections, development of respiratory tract pseudomonas colonization and infection, hemoptysis and pneumothorax, allergic bronchopulmonary aspergillosis, chronic cor pulmonale; hepatic cirrhosis; impaired fertility

Therapeutic Plan

nutritional support: pancreatic enzyme replacement, fat soluble vitamin replacement, increased caloric intake, careful monitoring of growth curves prevention and treatment of pulmonary disease: postural drainage and chest percussion, clinical trials using DNase to liquify sticky DNA-mucus complexes, influenza and pneumococcal vaccines, antibiotic therapy for 2-4 weeks with PO, IV, or inhaled drugs depending on severity of exacerbation, oxygen, bronchodilators, lung transplant

Prognosis

> 50% live to be 28-30 years of age

Asthma

Alternate Terminology

Hyper Reactive Airway Disease (HRAD) -- term often used but really a misnomer no universal definition of disease -- regarded as a diffuse, obstructive lung disease with
- hyperreaction of the airways to various stimuli
- a high degree of reversibility of the obstructive process with or without treatment

Epidemiology
- affects 10-15% of males and 7-10% of females sometime during childhood
- 80-90% of those with asthma will present before age 5
- most frequent admitting diagnosis of children's hospitals
- polygenic or multifactorial inheritance: a child with one parent with disease has a risk of 25%, this increases to 50-66% if both parents are affected

Pathophysiologic Abnormality
- hypersensitivity of the large and small airways to allergic and nonspecific stimuli resulting in release of chemical mediators from mast cells; resultant airway obstruction from bronchospasm, mucosal edema, and mucus production
- airway obstruction leads to nonuniform ventilation, hyperinflation, ventilation-perfusion mismatch, hypoxia, hypercarbia, acidosis, respiratory failure

Predisposing Conditions
- past mucosal injury (bronchopulmonary dysplasia, respiratory syncytial virus)
- family history
- presence of atopy in infant/child
- cigarette smoking in the home
- triggers for asthmatic attacks are specific for each individual

Symptoms

cough (nighttime cough, exercise-induced cough), wheezing, dyspnea

Physical Findings
- sometimes none--especially between attacks
- dry cough
- diffuse wheezing
- prolonged expiration
- use of accessory muscles of respiration
- retractions

Laboratory Findings

- Chest X-ray: hyperinflation, atelectasis
- ABGs: see chart - Progression of pH and Blood Gas Changes in Asthma in this chapter
  pulmonary function tests: bronchial provocation testing or pre- and post-bronchodilator measurements (increase at least 10% in peak flow rate or FEV1 is suggestive of asthma)

Potential Complications

- Psychological
  vulnerable child syndrome, limitation of physical activity, school absenteeism, social isolation
- Physical
  status asthmaticus, respiratory failure, pneumothorax, sudden death

Differential Diagnosis

bronchiolitis, cystic fibrosis, tracheomaleacia, pertussis, foreign body aspiration, congestive heart failure, intrathoracic tumor, gastroesophageal reflux

Therapeutic Plan

General Principles

- environmental control to avoid triggers
- monitoring of pulmonary function with peak flow meters and pulmonary function tests in older children
- use of spacers to aid in delivery of inhaled medication use of anti-inflammatory medications in children with chronic moderate to severe asthma with limitation of bronchodilators, if possible, to treat acute attacks

Pharmacologic

- bronchodilators (should be considered "rescue" drugs): beta-adrenergic drugs preferably by aerosols (albuterol, terbutaline, pirbuterol, metaproterenol) or orally (albuterol or theophylline), IV route may be used in status asthmaticus

- anti-inflammatory agents ("maintenance" drugs): **Cromolyn sodium**--prevents a degranulation of the mast cells, prevents exercise-induced bronchospasm in some patients, used daily to decrease inflammation advantages--no significant side effects, comes in inhaler and nebulizer form

- steroids--decrease airway hyperresponsiveness, decrease inflammation and mucosal edema
    * **Prednisone/prednisolone** orally for acute flareups (1-2mg/kg/24 hours for 5-7 days), may be given IV during hospitalization, IV and PO absorption similar
    * **Beclomethasone diproprionate, flunisolide,** and **triamcinolone** are available as inhalers; side effects in younger children may include immunologic suppression and decreased growth but neither have been convincingly proved, all are acceptable as an alternate drug in patients not controlled on cromolyn or in adolescent patients

Foreign Body Aspiration
Etiology
foreign body in the larynx, trachea or bronchus
Epidemiology
- 90% of deaths from foreign body aspiration occur in children < 5 years
- 50% of reported incidents occur in children < 2 years
- male-female ratio is 2:1
- commonly aspirated items include nuts, hot dogs, rattles, pacifiers, balloons, balls, and toy parts
Pathophysiologic Abnormality
- depends on the site of entrapment
- upper airway involvement may lead to complete obstruction, loss or abnormality of the voice
- obstruction of bronchus will result in atelectasis
- partial obstruction may cause emphysema, pneumothorax or pneumomediastinum through a "ball valve effect"
Predisposing Conditions
access of small objects to curious infants
Symptoms
- sudden onset of cough, dysphagia, stridor, dyspnea, cyanosis, choking; large percentage of patients have no acute symptoms
- classical triad: wheezing, cough and decreased breath sounds (absent in 50% of documented cases)

Physical Findings
>
> deviation of trachea; unilateral wheezing; localized decreased breath sounds; crackles; tachypnea

Laboratory Findings

- chest X-ray: mediastinal shift (toward lesion if atelectasis; away if ball valve obstruction)
- 25-33% will have normal X-ray
- subcutaneous air or pneumomediastinum; inspiratory and expiratory films may help identify ball valve effect

Differential Diagnosis
>
> see "Asthma" in this chapter

Therapeutic Plan

- total obstruction (aphonic and not breathing):
  > abdominal thrusts not used on infants--use four back blows followed by four chest compressions; "blind finger" sweeps not recommended
- symptoms dictate timing and nature of medical response: rigid bronchoscopy is the procedure of choice for removal

Jane E Puls

Developmental Considerations

Early Embryonic Development

By the time an embryo has an ovulation age of 21 days the vascular system has begun to appear as "blood islands", scattered masses of angiogenic cell clusters which increase in number and size, acquire a lumen and eventually form a vascular plexus. Part of the plexus differentiates in the main channels and, at the cephalad end of the embryo, these channels further specialize, producing a pair of heart tubes which come to lie parallel to each other and eventually fuse to form a single tube.

By 23 days of ovulation age differentiation continues into formation of the bulboventricular tube with an extra pericardial portion called the aortic sac. The cardiac loop forms and the caudal half of the bulboventricular tube begins to represent the early embryonic ventricle.

By an ovulation age of 25 days the heart completely occupies the pericardial cavity, while internally still a single tube but with primitive development of the left ventricle on the left side and the bulbos cordis on the right. A portion of the bulbos cordis eventually becomes the right ventricle.

Further development of the primitive atria and the truncus arteriosus occurs and by an ovulation age of about 27 days the external shape of the heart already suggests its future four chambered condition.

As the heart continues to develop, cardiac septation takes place, the ventricles enlarge in size, medial walls of the ventricles appose and fuse, forming the major portion of the muscular ventricular septum. The AV canal divides into a right and left atrioventricular orifice. Vascular structures change in their alignment and blood can begin to flow from one chamber to the other (an embryology text or specific book on the heart has further details on embryonic development).

As the heart continues development the pulmonary veins develop, along with the atrioventricular valves. Septums continue formation, the chordae tendineae are initially formed, arterial valves are formed and the cardiovascular system increases in size and complexity.

Early in embryonic development aortic arches form (1st, 2nd, 3rd, 4th, and 6th, (the 5th aortic arch is generally not present in humans or is very rudimentary)). Aortic arches progress through a complex series of transformations. **The ductus arteriosus in the prenatal child is the distal portion of the left 6th aortic arch. This obliterates after birth and is converted to the ligamentum arteriosum.**

Because the cardiovascular system in the fetus is required during fetal life for the supply of oxygenated blood to all tissues of the fetus, the cardiovascular system develops quite precociously. This results in complete organization of the cardiovascular system by an ovulation age of 8 weeks.

Fetal Circulation
The fetal circulation has some marked differences from circulation in the postnatal infant. Oxygenated blood is supplied to the fetal heart for distribution to the fetus from the placenta through the umbilical vein and has a PaO_2 of about 35mm Hg. Approximately 50% of this blood flows through the liver and the other 50% bypasses the liver through the ductus venosus into the inferior vena cava and to the right atrium. It then flows across the foramen ovale to the left atrium, into the left ventricle, and is ejected into the ascending aorta, from which it supplies the upper portion of the body. Blood returning through the superior vena cava flows through the right atrium and into the right ventricle, where it is ejected into the pulmonary arterial trunk. Most of this blood flows through the ductus arteriosus into the descending aorta and supplies the lower portion of the body. A small portion of this blood will flow through the pulmonary arteries to the lungs.

Pulmonary resistance is much higher in the fetus than in the newborn and accounts for blood preferentially crossing the ductus arteriosus and bypassing the lungs.

At birth fetal circulation stops and neonatal circulation begins. Changes that result in this include: an initial fall in systemic blood pressure followed by a progressive rise, a decrease in pulmonary vascular resistance with an increase in pulmonary blood flow, increased pulmonary venus return and left ventricular outflow, closure of the ductus arteriosus and the ductus venosus, and the formation of the ligamentum venosus and the ligamentum arteriosus. As well, the foramen ovale begins its apposition to the atrial wall and is functionally closed by 3 months of age.

Until the pulmonary vascular pressures decrease after birth to a level sufficiently below that of the systemic pressures, left to right flow will not occur through septal defects and the murmurs generated by such flow will not be heard. This means that many infants with VSDs, etc, will be undiagnosed during their newborn nursery stay and will present later. A thorough cardiovascular exam is imperative when evaluating infants.

Diagnostic Modalities

History
General history plus specific questioning about:
Cyanosis--resting
Blueness during exercise
Fatigue
Nocturnal dyspnea
Orthopnea
Failure to thrive or poor growth
Family history of congenital heart disease
Volume per feed
Dyspneic while sucking
Perspires profusely
Exhausted sleeping after feeds
Requires frequent feeds

Physical Examination
Growth and development
Length average and weight decreased
Tachypnea
Liver enlargement
Spleen enlargement
Crackles
Peripheral edema
Cyanosis
Clubbing
Cardiac rate - note normals for age
    Newborn 70 - 190
    Infant 80 - 160
    6 yrs. 75 - 115
    10 yrs. 70 - 110
    Adult   50 - 95
Character of the pulses

Blood pressure - varies by age, height, weight (also varies by exam; repeated measurements essential for reliability)

    Normal (after 1 year of age) can be approximated by:

        Systolic Blood Pressure = 70 + (age in years X 2)

        Diastolic Blood Pressure = 2/3 of systolic pressure

Cardiac examination

    Visual observation

        Hyperdynamic or silent precordium

        Precordial bulge

        Apical heave

        Substernal thrust

    Palpation

        Thrills

        Bruits

    Auscultation

        Heart sounds

            Characteristics

            Splitting

            Intensity

        Murmurs

        Clicks

        Rubs

Physical Examination Findings Suggestive of Heart Disease

Hepatomegaly	The neonate and infant rarely get pedal edema from CHF, but hepatomegaly is almost always present.
Cyanosis	3 to 5 g/dl of unsaturated Hgb is required to see cyanosis. Thus severe hypoxemia can be missed in patients who are anemic enough.
Precordial prominence	Reflective of long standing cardiomegaly during development of the chest wall.
Hyperdynamic precordium	Suggestive of extra volume (as in left-to-right shunts) if not in febrile children.
Any diastolic murmur	Diastolic murmurs should not be heard in normal healthy children.

Heart Murmurs

Grades of Murmurs

Grade	I	Soft heard only with difficulty
Grade	II	Easily heard
Grade	III	Loud but without a palpable thrill on the chest wall
Grade	IV	Loud with a palpable thrill
Grade	V	Heard with only one edge of the stethoscope on the chest
Grade	VI	Heard without the stethoscope touching the chest

Cardiac Cycle Location of Murmurs

Systole - Murmurs heard between the first heart sound (S_1) and the second heart sound (S_2).

Systolic Ejection Murmur (SEM)

There is a silent interval between S_1 and the onset of the murmur. It then crescendos to a maximum intensity and decrescendos to end before the S_2 heart sound. These murmurs arise in stenotic aortic or pulmonary valve areas and must overcome the pressure in such vessels before the flow rate is great enough to produce a murmur.

Holosystolic Murmur

Also called pansystolic murmurs, these are the result of immediate flow from a high pressure area to a low flow area and are heard throughout systole. Areas of such pressure differentials are from a ventricle to an atrium, or from the left ventricle to the right ventricle.

End Systolic Murmur

Also called late systolic murmurs, these murmurs are caused by prolapse of the mitral valve toward the end of systole, allowing regurgitation of blood into the left atrium.

Diastole - Murmurs heard between the second heart sound (S_2) and the first heart sound (S_1).

Early Diastolic Murmur

Murmurs beginning with S_2 are due to back-flow through incompetent outflow tract valves and are generated by pressure in the aorta or pulmonary vessels. They rarely can be heard beyond mid diastole. Characteristically they are high-pitched blowing murmurs.

Mid Diastolic Murmur

These murmurs are the result of turbulent flow over the mitral or tricuspid valves during the atrial filling phase of diastole. They are due to either an actual or relative (increased volume over normal-sized valves) flow across these valves. These are usually very low-pitched rumbling murmurs.

Late Diastolic Murmur

These are the result of end diastolic filling into a ventricle with decreased compliance, as occurs in ventricular hypertrophy. These may sound more like a click than a distinct murmur.

Continuous

Continuous murmurs continue through S_2. They begin in late systole and continue in early diastole. A typical continuous murmur is that of a PDA. The systolic component is due to increased flow across a relatively stenotic pulmonary valve and the diastolic component is generated by the flow through the ductus from the aorta to the pulmonary vessel at the beginning of diastole.

Point of Maximal Intensity of Murmurs, Typical

Aortic area: 2nd right intercostal space (ICS)
Pulmonary area: 2nd left intercostal space
Mitral area: the cardiac apex
Tricuspid area: left lower sternal border (LSB)

Pitch Qualities of Murmurs

Blowing: high pitched.
This sound can be simulated by holding the stethoscope in the palm and stroking then back of the hand with the pad of a finger.

Harsh: medium pitched.
This sound can be simulated by holding the stethoscope in the palm and scratching the back of the hand with a fingernail.

Rumbling: low pitched.
This is the sound of a bowling ball rumbling down a gutter.

Characteristics of Murmurs in Selected Heart Lesions

Lesion	Loudest	Quality	Radiation
Aortic stenosis	Right 3rd ICS	Harsh, SEM	Carotids
Aortic regurgitation	MLSB	Blowing, early diastolic	Apex
Pulmonary stenosis	Left 2nd ICS	Harsh, SEM	Lung fields
Pulmonary regurgitation	Left 2nd ICS	Low pitched, early-mid diastolic	Little to none
Mitral stenosis	Apex	Low pitched, mid diastolic rumble	None
Mitral regurgitation	Apex	Blowing, holosystolic	Left axilla
ASD	Left 2nd ICS	Harsh, SEM	Lung fields
VSD	LLSB	Harsh, holosystolic	None
PDA	Left 2nd - 3rd ICS	Continuous	Lung fields

Characteristics of Functional (Still's) Murmurs

- Systolic ejection murmur
- Grade III or less
- Vibratory quality
- Non radiating

Remember that innocent murmurs are uncommon in the newborn, except for physiologic peripheral pulmonic stenosis.

Chest X-ray - Note size of heart and amount of pulmonary blood flow (heart size normally occupies 50% or less of the chest and pulmonary vessels are seen from the hilar area throughout 2/3 of the chest).

Electrocardiogram - Shows myocardial mass as it is reflected by electrical activity seen at the surface and shows cardiac rhythm.

> NOTE: As a result of fetal circulation, the newborn heart has a relative right ventricular hypertrophy. The muscle mass of the right ventricle is roughly equal to the mass of the left ventricle. Postnatally the left ventricular muscle mass begins to increase and gradually the relative right ventricular hypertrophy resolves.

> Most children's heart disease is "structural" rather than the "functional" heart disease seen in adults. Children's hearts are generally, if you will, "malformed" rather than "malfunctioning". These diseases are reflected in different ways in the electrocardiogram (see under disease profiles).

Echocardiography - Forms available now include M-mode and two-dimensional echocardiography, as well as pulsed continuous wave and color-flow doppler. These forms now give precise information about cardiac structure and blood flow and are an essential adjunct in evaluation of the patient **when done by an experienced echocardiographer with interpretation by a pediatric cardiologist.**

A relatively new method of using echocardiography is esophageal echo. In special circumstances in children, such as anomalous return, this can be a valuable tool.

Echocardiography is an incredibly versatile tool for prenatal diagnosis of both structural and functional congenital heart disease. It should be routinely included as a part of the prenatal ultrasound.

Exercise Testing - Used most commonly in patients with known heart disease to assess effective exercise on cardiac function, as a guide to prescribing activity for the child.
Most helpful in children with:
Arrhythmias
Chronic volume overload of the ventricles
Left ventricular outflow obstruction
Hypertension

Radionuclide Studies - A relatively non-invasive procedure that can be used to assess blood flow, shunts, etc; also available on a portable basis. Does not provide the information about anatomic details provided by echocardiography and catheterization, but may be useful in some patients.

166

Cardiac Catheterization - Always a good tool for delineation of anatomy and understanding of directional flow in an individual's heart, the cardiac cath is used less frequently since the advent of echocardiography. However, it remains a good tool for this purpose and an essential tool for the measurement of PaO_2, etc. in the various chambers of the heart. This information may be necessary for planning corrective surgery, etc. for a child.

Laboratory Data - Some or all of these may be appropriate depending on the patient's particular situation. Patients who are polycythemic as a result of their heart disease frequently have other hematologic abnormalities.
    Arterial blood gas
    Serum chemistries
    Complete blood count
    Frequent follow-up of hemoglobin and hematocrit
    Platelet count
    Fibrinogen level
    PT/PTT

Pathophysiologic Manifestations

Supraventricular tachycardia in the neonate and infant is often initially mistakenly diagnosed as sepsis.

Only 40 - 50% of CHD (Congenital Heart Disease) is diagnosed by one week of age. Only 50 - 60% of CHD is diagnosed by one month of age.

Incidence of CHD is 10 times higher in stillborn than in live born infants.

Incidence of CHD in stillborns plus spontaneous abortions plus live borns is five times that of the incidence of CHD in live borns alone.

Incidence in the live born child of CHD is approximately 1% (varies from .4 - 1.0 depending on the study). This number is probably an underestimation.

It is felt that most estimates underrepresent CHD because the majority of the studies that estimates are based on were done when echocardiography was not available, and some things (like bicuspid aortic valve, occurs in approximately 2% of the population) are best diagnosed with echocardiography.

Risk for recurrence - this is impossible to predict in the overall sense, partly because it is different for specific lesions. In general, the recurrence risk is higher if the proband has a more serious lesion, if the affected parent is the mother, or if more than one first degree relative is affected. Recurrence risk for siblings is approximately 2 - 3%. Transmission risk to next generation is approximately 5 - 10%.

Common chromosomal abnormalities associated with CHD (chromosomal defects account for 5 - 8% of CHD):

Single gene defects - account for 3% of CHD.
    Autosomal dominant:
        Marfan's - aortic and mitral valve incompetence, dilatation of the ascending aorta.
        Holt-Oram - VSD, ASD
        Noonan's - PS, ASD, cardiomyopathy
    Autosomal recessive:
        Pompe (Type II-A glycogen storage disease) - cardiomyopathy
        Ellis-van Creveld - single atrium
    X-linked:
        Duchenne Muscular Dystrophy - cardiomyopathy

Polygenic inheritance.
    Well-described for PDA with a recurrence risk of 2.5% in siblings (recurrence risk increased to 10% if > than one family member affected).

Some CHDs are more common in one sex than the other:
    AS - more common in males
    Coarctation - more common in males
    ASD - more common in females
    PDA - more common in females
    VSD - equal in both sexes

The most common form of CHD is VSD (30 - 40% of all CHD).

Congenital Syndromes Associated with Congenital Heart Disease

Syndrome	Heart Lesion
• Trisomy 13	VSD, ASD, PDA
• Trisomy 18	VSD, ASD, PDA
• Trisomy 21	Endocardial cushion defect
• Turner syndrome	Coarctation of the aorta, aortic stenosis
• Williams syndrome	Supravalvular aortic stenosis
• Noonan syndrome	Pulmonary valve stenosis, aortic valve stenosis
• Holt-Oram syndrome	ASD, VSD
• Marfan syndrome	Mitral valve prolapse, aortic valve regurgitation, dilated and dissecting aorta
• Asplenia syndrome	Complex cyanotic heart lesions, anomalous pulmonary venous return, dextrocardia, single ventricle, single AV valve
• Polysplenia syndrome	Pulmonary atresia, dextrocardia, single ventricle, azygos continuation of inferior vena cava
• Congenital rubella	PDA, peripheral pulmonic stenosis
• Glycogen storage disease	Hypertrophic cardiomyopathy
• DiGeorge syndrome	Aortic arch anomalies, Tetralogy of Fallot, pulmonary atresia, transposition of great vessels, truncus arteriosus

Association	Heart Lesion
• CHARGE association Coloboma Heart lesion Atresia of choanae Retardation Genital anomalies Ear anomalies	Tetralogy of Fallot, endocardial cushion defects, VSD, ASD
• VATER association Vertebral anomalies Anal atresia Tracheo esophageal fistula Esophageal atresia Radial and renal anomalies	VSD

Acyanotic Congenital Heart Lesions

With increased pulmonary blood flow (vascularity) [left-to-right shunts]
- Arterial septal defect
- Patent ductus arteriosus
- Ventricular septal defect
- Endocardial cushion defect
- Arteriovenous malformation

With normal pulmonary blood flow [no left-to-right shunt]
- Coarctation
- Aortic stenosis
- Pulmonary stenosis (without right-to-left shunt)
- Mitral stenosis
- Mitral regurgitation
- Endocardial fibroelastosis

Cyanotic Congenital Heart Lesions

With decreased pulmonary flow (vascularity) [pulmonary outflow obstruction]
- Pulmonary stenosis
- Pulmonary atresia
- Tetralogy of Fallot
- Tricuspid atresia
- Pulmonary atresia and hypoplastic right ventricle
- Ebstein anomaly

With increased pulmonary blood flow
- Hypoplastic left heart syndrome
- Total anomalous pulmonary venous return
- Transposition of great vessels
- Single ventricle complexes
- Truncus arteriosus

Common Causes of Heart Failure By Age

Fetus
- Severe anemia
- Supraventricular tachycardia
- Ventricular tachycardia
- Complete block

Premature Infant
- Cardiomyopathy from asphyxia, sepsis, hypoglycemia, hypocalcemia
- Fluid overload
- PDA
- VSD
- Cor pulmonale from BPD

Term Infant
- Cardiomyopathy from asphyxia, sepsis, hypoglycemia, hypocalcemia
- A-V malformation (vein of Galen, hepatic)
- Left-sided obstructive lesions (hypoplastic left heart, coarctation of aorta)
- Large mixing cardiac defects (single ventricle, truncus arteriosus)
- Viral myocarditis

Infant-Toddler
- Left-to-right cardiac shunts (VSD)
- Hemangioma (arteriovenous malformation)
- Anomalous left coronary artery
- Metabolic cardiomyopathy
- Acute hypertension (hemolytic-uremic syndrome)
- Supraventricular tachycardia
- Coronary aa. aneurysms (Kawasaki disease)

Child-Adolescent
- Rheumatic fever
- Acute hypertension
- Viral myocarditis
- Thyrotoxicosis
- Hemochromatosis-hemosiderosis
- Cancer therapy (radiation, adriamycin)
- Sickle-cell anemia
- Endocarditis
- Cor pulmonale (cystic fibrosis)
- Status asthmaticus

Therapeutic Considerations

Lesions Amenable to Prostaglandin (PGE₁) Palliation

Hypoplastic left heart syndrome
Complex coarctation syndromes
Critical aortic stenosis
Hypoplastic right heart syndrome
  Pulmonary atresia with intact ventricular septum
  Tricuspid atresia
Pulmonary atresia with VSD

Mneumonic for Treating CHF/Pulmonary Edema

		Mechanism of Action
U	Upright position	Improve ventilation-perfusion
N	Nifedipine, nitroglycerine, nitroprusside	Afterload reduction
L	Lasix	Diuresis, fluid shift
O	Oxygen	Improved O_2 saturation
A	Albuterol inhalation	Bronchodilation
D	Dopamine, dobutamine, digitalis	Inotropic agents
M	Morphine	Anxiolytic, venous pooling
E	Extremity tourniquets	Decrease preload

Surgical Procedures for Selected CHD Lesions

Palliative Procedures

Procedure	Anatomy Involved	Result	Indication
Blalock-Taussig shunt	subclavian artery to ipsilateral pulmonary artery	increased pulmonary blood flow	tetralogy of Fallot pulmonary valve atresia
Modified Blalock-Taussig shunt	tube graft from subclavian artery to ipsilateral PA	increased pulmonary blood flow	tetralogy of Fallot pulmonary valve atresia
Waterston shunt	aorta to right pulmonary artery	increased pulmonary blood flow	tetralogy of Fallot pulmonary valve atresia tricuspid atresia
Rashkind procedure	balloon atrial septostomy	increased atrial mixing	transposition of great arteries
		decompression of right or left atria	tricuspid atresia
Blalock-Hanlon procedure	operative arterial septostomy	increased atrial mixing	transposition of great arteries
		decompression of right or left atria	tricuspid atresia
Balloon angioplasty	valves and vessels	dilation of valves/ vessels	pulmonary valve stenosis aortic valve stenosis coarctation of the aorta
Pulmonary artery banding	pulmonary artery	decreased pulmonary blood flow and pressure	VSD endocardial cushion defect single ventricle

Palliative Procedures (Continued)

Procedure	Anatomy Involved	Result	Indication
Glenn shunt	superior vena cava to right pulmonary artery	increased pulmonary blood flow	used as a staging procedure prior to Fontan operation

Corrective Procedures

Procedure	Anatomy Involved	Result	Indication
Fontan procedure	right atrium or vena cava to pulmonary artery anastamosis	diverts systemic venous return directly to pulmonary circulation	tricuspid atresia single ventricle - pulmonary atresia
Mustard procedure (atrial switch)	intra-atrial baffle	RV remains systemic ventricle	transposition of great arteries (procedure rarely used)
Norwood procedure	pulmonary artery becomes ascending aorta	use right ventricle to pump to aorta	hypoplastic left heart
Heart transplant			hypoplastic left heart cardiomyopathy
Jatene procedure (arterial switch)	switch great arteries above the valve	anatomic correction	transposition of great arteries (replacing Mustard)

Disease Profiles

Only diseases that are common, specifically unique or important, or particularly interesting are included. A textbook has more comprehensive information.

Persistent Fetal Circulation
Not necessarily classified as a congenital heart disease, but typically occurs in the neonatal full term infant. Presents much like cyanotic congenital heart disease.

Alternate Terminology
PFC

Etiology
Uncertain in some cases, but most commonly related to perinatal hypoxemia.

Pathophysiology
Generally persistent pulmonary hypertension which results in left-to-right shunting through the foramen ovale and/or the patent ductus arteriosus.

Predisposing Conditions
Hypoxic insult at birth.

Symptoms
Tachypnea in the first few hours of life with varying degrees of respiratory distress.

Physical Examination
Ill appearance, +/- systolic murmur, +/- a loud second heart sound, +/- parasternal heave.

Laboratory Findings
Acidosis, X-ray with decreased vascular flow, echo with right-to-left flow seen at the foramen ovale.

Differential Diagnosis
Includes the cyanotic congenital heart diseases, most specifically transposition of the great arteries.

Potential Complications
Almost universally fatal if not treated, and even when treated has significant mortality.

Diagnostic Plan
Diagnosis based on physical exam plus X-ray, greatly helped by echocardiography and measurement of differential PaO_2s.

Therapeutic Plan

Oxygen administration, mechanical ventilation, correction of acidosis and any electrolyte abnormalities, administration of Tolazoline and consideration of possible use of ECMO (Extra Corporeal Membrane Oxygenation).

Congenital Structural Lesions

Hypoplastic Left-Heart Syndrome

Pathophysiologic Abnormality

Underdevelopment of the aortic root, aortic valve, left ventricle or mitral valve. Either or both valves may be atretic. Systemic flow is duct dependent.

Symptoms

Severe CHF and cardiovascular collapse occur as the duct closes.

Physical Findings

Signs of poor peripheral perfusion (mottling of skin, prolonged capillary refill, diminished or absent pulses) and congestive failure. A nonspecific murmur may be present.

Laboratory Findings

X-ray: cardiomegaly, pulmonary congestion

EKG: normal for age

ECHO: is diagnostic

Chronologic Sequence of Manifestations

Failure occurs early as the duct begins to close in the first few days or weeks of life.

Differential Diagnosis

Critical aortic stenosis, severe coarctation of aorta

Therapeutic Plan

Prostaglandin E_1, supportive care

Norwood procedure may allow survival through infancy

Transplant is corrective care

Hypoplastic Right-Heart Syndrome

Alternate Terminology

Either of the following can cause this syndrome:

Pulmonary atresia with intact ventricular septum

Tricuspid atresia with a patent ASD

Pathophysiologic Abnormality

Pulmonary perfusion is dependent on a patent ductus arteriosus in pulmonary atresia

Symptoms

Severe cyanosis at birth

Physical Findings

A continuous PDA murmur may be heard in the pulmonary atresia defect

Laboratory Findings

Chest X-ray: diminished pulmonary vascularity; variable heart size

EKG: right atrial enlargement; left axis deviation in tricuspid atresia

ECHO: is diagnostic

Chronologic Sequence of Manifestations

Rapid deterioration as the ductus closes

Differential Diagnosis

Severe pulmonary stenosis, Tetralogy of Fallot

Therapeutic Plan

Prostaglandin E_1, supportive care

Surgical establishment of an aorto-pulmonary artery shunt

Atrial Septal Defect

The most common CHD found in **adults** (discounting congenital bicuspid aortic valve).

Alternate Terminology

ASD, Ostium Premum Defect, Ostium Secundum (Defect at the Fossa Ovalis)

Predisposing Conditions

More common in females, with 2 to 1 ratio, female to male. Genetics multifactorial, but some Mendelian examples available.

Symptoms

Usually asymptomatic, may have mild fatigue. If persists uncorrected into adulthood, may develop fatigue, dyspnea, chest pain, etc.

Physical Findings

Growth and development usually normal, +/-right ventricular systolic lift, +/- accentuated first heart sound, plus fixed splitting of second heart sound, plus systolic murmur at LUSB.

Laboratory Findings

CXR - Some heart enlargement, prominence of pulmonary vasculature.

EKG - Regular sinus rhythm pattern.

ECHO - Shows left-to-right shunt with resultant right-sided volume overload. Sometimes (usually) can visualize and categorize actual defect.

Cath - Increased O_2 saturation in right side of heart.

Chronologic Sequence of Manifestations

Few findings early in life, so many individuals not diagnosed until adulthood. As adults, may develop pulmonary hypertension and congestive heart failure or atrial arrhythmias.

Differential Diagnosis

Valvular - competent foramen ovale.

Potential Complications

Pulmonary hypertension, congestive heart failure, atrial fibrillation or flutter, mitral valve prolapse, infections.

Diagnostic Plan

Usually murmur noted on routine exam leads to chest x-ray, EKG, ECHO, and possibly catheterization.

Therapeutic Plan

Watchful waiting in younger children with elective repair prior to school age. Repair adults. Repair is usually direct repair or patch repair of defect. Genetic counseling about inheritance.

Ventricular Septal Defect

Alternate Terminology

VSD

Etiology

Prenatal incomplete development of the ventricular septum.

Pathophysiology

Depends on the size of the defect. Small defects have high resistance to flow across the defect, with little resultant shunting. Moderate defects have significant left-to-right shunting, with much higher pressures in the left ventricle than the right. Large defects have relatively complete mixing of the blood in the ventricles, with right ventricular pressure equal to left.

Symptoms

Depends on the size of the defect. Small - asymptomatic. Large - congestive failure symptoms (sweating, tachypnea, grunting respirations, fatigue with feeds).

Physical Findings

Systolic murmur, +/- LLSB thrill. Children with large defects have respiratory distress, decreased weight for height, narrowly split S^2, hepatomegaly.

Laboratory Findings

CXR - Small defect - normal. Large defect - enlarged heart with prominent pulmonary vascular markings.

EKG - Large defect - QRS axis oriented to the right, bilaterally increased ventricular voltage, increased left atrial voltage.

ECHO - Images defect. Invaluable.

Cath - Reflection of left-to-right shunt found in increased O_2 saturation of blood in right ventricle.

Chronologic Sequence of Manifestations

Most small isolated VSDs are insignificant and close spontaneously. Large VSDs +/- other defects progress to congestive failure with pulmonary damage.

Diagnostic Plan

Diagnosis based on physical exam plus X-ray and ECHO. ECHO demonstrates not only size and location of defect, but blood flow across defect.

Therapeutic Plan

Surgical repair of moderate or large defects. Most small defects are followed with repeat exams and close spontaneously.

Atrioventricular Canal Defect

Atrioventricular canals are generally described in two basic types:

Partial (comprised of ostium premum atrial septal defect, cleft mitral valve and deficient ventricular septum, but without significant interventricular shunting.)

Complete (Atrial septal defect, essentially single valve from atria to ventricles comprised of tissue of mitral and tricuspid valves, and deficient ventricular septum with shunting.)

Complete form much less common and much more severe than partial form. About half of children with Down syndrome have congenital heart disease, and a large percentage of this is the atrioventricular canal.

Alternate Terminology

AV Canal, Endocardial Cushion Defect

Etiology

Incomplete growth of the endocardial cushions.

Pathophysiology

Atrial septal defect of the lower part of the septum, cleft mitral valve +/- cleft tricuspid valve and inadequate tissue of the ventricular septum.

Associated Conditions

Nearly all patients with Asplenia syndrome have a complete atrioventricular canal. Other associated conditions include: Tetralogy of Fallot, polysplenia, disorder of right ventricle, Down syndrome.

Symptoms

Depends on type: Partial have symptoms similar to patients with simple atrial septal defect unless their mitral valve is compromised to the point that they have significant mitral regurg. Then they are likely to have fatigue, dyspnea, failure to gain weight adequately, repeated respiratory infections, etc. Those with complete atrioventricular canals progress rapidly to congestive heart failure and generally do very poorly without corrective surgery.

Physical Findings

Partial: +/- systolic murmur at LUSB, +/-holosystolic blowing, murmur at the apex. Complete: plus systolic murmur at LUSB, plus systolic murmur at LLSB, plus fixed splitting of second heart sound, +/- hepatomegaly and evidence of congestive heart failure.

Laboratory Findings

CXR - Cardiac enlargement +/- pulmonary congestion

EKG - Superior orientation of the mean QRS axis in the frontal plane, +/- prolonged QT interval.

ECHO - Visualization of atrial septal defect, valvular function, ventricular septal defect with evaluation of shunt, and evaluation of ventricular size and ability that may influence surgical plans.

Cath - Increased O_2 saturation in right atrium, increased right ventricular pressure (in complete type).

Chronologic Sequence of Manifestations

Partial defects progress as atrial septal defects with an increased risk of infection 2° to mitral valve deformity. Complete defects usually progress rapidly to congestive heart failure and die if not corrected in some fashion.

Differential Diagnosis

Must distinguish from simple atrial septal defect, simple ventricular septal defect, and must delineate type.

Potential Complications

High risk of endocardial infection with valvular disease, many children (especially with complete atrioventricular canal) have associated disease.

Diagnostic Plan

Diagnose with high level of suspicion (Asplenia syndrome, Down syndrome), history, physical, especially EKG and ECHO.

Therapeutic Plan

Medical management in those with fewer symptoms, surgical correction in those with significant mitral regurg or complete atrioventricular canal. Small infants may require pulmonary banding (to decrease pressure to lung fields) until at an age where surgical correction is possible.

Patent Ductus Arteriosus
    Alternate Terminology
        PDA
    Etiology
        Failure of the ductus arteriosus to close after birth
    Pathophysiologic Abnormality
        The direction of flow through the duct is dependent on the relative pressures in the systemic and pulmonary circuits, it can be either left-to-right or visa versa.
    Predisposing Conditions
        prematurity
    Symptoms
        Large left-to-right shunts can result in failure to thrive, CHF; right-to-left shunts cause dyspnea and cyanosis
    Physical Findings
        Bounding pulses are characteristic of large left-to-right shunts
        A continuous murmur is present after the pulmonary pressure decreases enough for a large shunt to occur
    Laboratory Findings
        Chest X-ray: cardiomegaly and increased pulmonary vascularity in large left-to-right shunts
        EKG: biventricular hypertrophy; right ventricular hypertrophy indicates development of increased pulmonary resistance
    Potential Complications
        Pulmonary hypertension
    Therapeutic Plan
        Surgical ligation or coil ablation of the duct before pulmonary hypertension develops
    Prognosis
        Good if corrected. If pulmonary hypertension develops (usually after a year), it is irreversible

Congenital Mitral Stenosis
Commonly associated with PDA, AS, coarc.
    Etiology
        Malformed mitral valve, funnel-shaped, with thickened leaflets and short, deformed cordae tendineae.
    Symptoms
        Underdeveloped infants with dyspnea 2° to CHF.
        Cyanosis
        Pallor

Physical Findings

Rumbling diastolic murmur followed by a loud first sound. Second sound split and loud.

Laboratory Findings

EKG - RVH

X-ray - Left atrial and right ventricular enlargement, pulmonary congestion.

ECHO - Enlarged left atrium, thick mitral valve leaflets.

Therapeutic Plan

Poor prognosis. Mitral valve prothesis. Usually die early.

Aortic Stenosis

Etiology

Congenital (usually bicuspid); acquired in Rheumatic fever; or part of Williams syndrome

Pathophysiologic Abnormality

Outflow obstruction to the left ventricle

Symptoms

Most patients are asymptomatic until adulthood when syncope, easy fatiguability or anginal pain may occur

Physical Findings

Harsh systolic ejection murmur at right 2nd ICS, radiating to carotids; systolic thrill at jugular notch

Laboratory Findings

Chest X-ray: Post-stenotic dilatation of aorta

EKG: left ventricular hypertrophy

ECHO: identifies the lesion and location

Therapeutic Plan

Bacterial endocarditis prophylaxis; surgical repair if severity warrants

Coarctation of the Aorta

Pathophysiologic Abnormality

Narrowing of the aorta, most commonly at level of the ductus arteriosus

Predisposing Conditions

- Male sex
- Turner syndrome in females

Symptoms

Coarctation generally presents in one of three ways. Because of the position of the ductus in relation to the usual coarctation, as long as the ductus remains open in the newborn, infants are asymptomatic. If the ductus closes early enough an infant may be diagnosed with coarctation in the newborn nursery based on the finding of absent femoral pulses. Many infants will leave the nursery without their diagnosis being made. A certain percent of these infants will have significant enough coarctation that they will proceed to heart failure in the first month of life. These infants usually present at about two weeks of age with the symptoms of heart failure with poor perfusion and "shocky" appearance. They require emergent care of their disease and usually emergent surgical correction. Many patients with coarctation of the aorta remain asymptomatic throughout childhood. Their coarctation may be found incidentally on well-child exam for sports physicals, etc.

Physical Findings

As noted under symptoms the physical findings depend largely on the time that the coarctation is diagnosed in the child. Diminished or absent femoral pulses is always a clue and checking peripheral pulses remains an important part of the cardiovascular exam of the child. Occasionally a child presents who has a small shoe size for age as a clue to their coarctation and hypertension can be a physical finding in long-standing coarct.

Laboratory Findings

- Chest X-ray: rib notching (> 5 years old), abnormal aortic knob
- EKG: may show LVH if severe and prolonged
- ECHO: sometimes can visualize the lesion
- MRI: may allow very good delineation of the lesion preoperatively and can be used for follow-up visualization after repairs.
  NOTE: Patient's who had patch corrections of coarctation done years ago may develop post-op complication of an aneurysm (particularly females during pregnancy) MRI can be very useful for this diagnosis.

Chronologic Sequence of Manifestations

About 10% develop CHF in infancy

Therapeutic Plan

- Bacterial endocarditis prophylaxis is indicated
- Repair should be undertaken either with balloon angioplasty or with a graft or patch surgical repair

Pulmonary Stenosis
Pathophysiologic Abnormality
Cyanosis results from decreased pulmonary perfusion, and in severe stenosis with increased right atrial pressure, from a right-to-left shunt through the foramen ovale. Peripheral pulmonary stenosis is a different lesion associated with congenital rubella syndrome.
Symptoms
Most are asymptomatic
Physical Findings
Cyanosis, if severe; systolic ejection murmur at 2nd left ICS radiating into posterior lung fields
Laboratory Findings
Chest X-ray: decreased pulmonary vascularity and cardiomegaly if the stenosis is severe
EKG: degree of right axis deviation correlates with severity of stenosis
Therapeutic Plan
Bacterial endocarditis prophylaxis
Surgical repair or balloon angioplasty if severity warrants

Tetralogy of Fallot
Most common **cyanotic** congenital heart lesion
Pathophysiologic Abnormality
- Right ventricular outflow obstruction (pulmonary stenosis)
- Dextroposition of aorta (overrides the ventricular septum)
- Ventricular septal defect
- Right ventricular hypertrophy
The degree of right ventricular outflow obstruction governs the degree of hypoxemia and right-to-left shunt.
Physical Findings
Cyanosis; harsh holosystolic murmur at LSB; squatting posture; exertional dyspnea
Laboratory Findings
Chest X-ray: Boot-shaped normal size heart; decreased pulmonary vascularity; may have right-sided aortic arch
EKG: right axis deviation, RVH
ECHO: is diagnostic
Potential Complications
Hypercyanotic spells (Tet spells)

Therapeutic Plan
> Bacterial endocarditis prophylaxis
> Surgical palliation: Blalock-Taussig procedure, modified Blalock-Taussig
> > procedure
> Definitive surgical repair

Persistent Truncus Arteriosus
Pathophysiologic Abnormality
> Single trunk from the heart; pulmonary arteries arise from this trunk; a
> large VSD is present

Physical Findings
> Findings relate to size of pulmonary artery and may resemble either a PDA
> or Tetralogy of Fallot

Laboratory Findings
> ECHO: is diagnostic

Therapeutic Plan
> Surgical repair may be done

D-Transposition of the Great Arteries
Alternate Terminology
> Simple transposition of the great vessels

Pathophysiologic Abnormality
> Pulmonary and systemic blood are recirculated through their own circuits;
> a communication between the circuits (ASD, VSD, PDA) must exist for
> survival

Predisposing Conditions
> More common in males

Physical Findings
> Cyanosis is present at birth

Laboratory Findings
> Chest X-ray: egg-on-a-string appearance of heart

Chronologic Sequence of Manifestations
> CHF develops early if surgical communication between the two circuits is
> not created

Therapeutic Plan
> Balloon atrial septostomy (Rashkin procedure) may be lifesaving; surgical
> correction can be done later. This usually involves the Jatene procedure.

L-Transposition of the Great Arteries
    Alternate Terminology
        Corrected transposition of the great vessels
    Pathophysiologic Abnormality
        There are usually associated anomalies which determine the exact nature of this complex lesion for any individual patient.

Total Anomalous Pulmonary Venous Return
    Alternate Terminology
        TAPVR
    Pathogenesis
        Common pulmonary vein does not get incorporated into the posterior wall of the left atrium
    Pathophysiologic Abnormality
        Pulmonary venous return is not to the left atrium but instead to one or a combination of the following routes:
            Supracardiac (into the innominate vein)
            Cardiac (into the coronary sinus or back to the right atrium)
            Infracardiac (infradiaphragmatic-into the inferior vena cava)
        Each of these lesions must have a right-to-left shunt, usually via the foramen ovale; pulmonary venous obstruction is often present and its degree determines the degree of cyanosis present.
    Laboratory Findings
        Chest X-ray: typical "snowman" or figure 8 heart shape
    Therapeutic Plan
        Surgical reimplantation of the veins into the left atrium

Partial Anomalous Pulmonary Venous Return
    Alternate Terminology
        PAPVR
    Pathophysiology
        One or more of the pulmonary veins returns to the right atrium instead of to the left atrium, sometimes associated with an atrial septal defect.
    Symptoms
        Depends on number of veins with anomalous connection. Single vein, usually asymptomatic. Multiple veins, symptoms of fatigue and dyspnea.
    Physical Findings
        +/- right ventricular systolic lift, plus widely split (but not fixed splitting) of second heart sound.

Laboratory Findings

CXR - Some enlargement of right side of heart, increased pulmonary vasculature.

EKG - +/- evidence of right volume overload.

ECHO - Plus increase right-sided flow seen, +/- visualization of anomalous vein(s).

Cath - May be able to directly enter anomalous veins and visualize return with contrast.

Chronologic Sequence of Manifestations

Depends on number of anomalous veins. Increased return to right side of heart leads to congestive heart failure.

Therapeutic Plan

In patients with large right-sided return, large right-to-left shunts through associated atrial septal defects or pulmonary hypertension with congestive heart failure, surgical correction is required.

Acquired Structural Lesions

Kawasaki Disease

Not truly a "heart" disease, this is a rheumatic disease with "heart" sequelae.

Etiology

Unknown, but a viral etiology is strongly suspected based on cyclic occurrence and seasonal occurrence (winter and spring).

Pathophysiology

Inflammation ($\uparrow$ lymphocytes and cytokines) with endothelial damage

Predisposing Conditions

Japanese ancestry; young age (85% of cases are in children < 5 years)

Diagnosis

Kawasaki's occurs in three phases and has specific criteria for diagnosis (five of six criteria needed for diagnosis). The acute phase (~10 days) includes conjunctivitis, fever, rash, changes in oral mucous membranes. The subacute phases (~ days 11-21) usually has decrease in fever, arthritis and skin desquamation. The convalescent phase may have thrombocytosis and arthritis and is generally when the development of coronary aa. aneurysms is seen.

Criteria for Diagnosis

- Mucosal changes (strawberry tongue, erythematous lips, general oral mucosal injection)
- Cervical lymphadenopathy
- Rash

- Extremity changes
  * Initial stage - erythema of palms and soles
  * Convalescent stage - desquamation

Differential Diagnosis
- Erythema multiform
- Measles
- Drug reaction
- Scarlet fever
- Scaled skin syndrome
- Juvenile rheumatoid arthritis

Potential Complications

Coronary artery aneurysms, with possibility of stenosis, thrombosis, and infarct; pericarditis, myocarditis

NOTE: Males < 1 year of age have a very high rate of coronary aa. aneurysms

Therapeutic Plan

Early diagnosis with administration of high-dose gamma globulin

Acquired Functional Diseases

Rheumatic Fever
   Pathogenesis

Unknown, related to an immune reaction to untreated group A beta-hemolytic streptococcus infection.

   Predisposing Conditions

More common in children 5-15, but can occur at all ages, though rarely in infancy (group A strep infections rare in infants)

   Diagnosis

Based on clinical presentation. Criteria developed years ago called Jones system include:

Major Criteria	Minor Criteria
• Polyarthritis	• Fever
• Carditis	• Arthralgias
• Chorea	• Elevated ESR/CRP
• Subcutaneous nodules	• Prolonged PR interval

Diagnosis requires the finding of two major or one major and two minor criteria along with documentation of a recent streptococcal infection.

Potential Complications

Patients who develop chronic rheumatic heart disease may develop mitral regurgitation, mitral stenosis, a combination of mitral stenosis and mitral regurgitation or aortic regurgitation with or without aortic stenosis.

Therapeutic Plan

- Aspirin in anti-inflammatory doses
- Prophylactic antibiotic therapy (oral or parenteral)
- Symptomatic care of children with bed rest, etc

Arteriosclerosis

Arteriosclerosis and coronary artery disease are rare in infants and children but as our nation becomes more obese and less active these diseases are being seen in a steadily younger population.

Predisposing Conditions

- Positive family history of heart attacks or strokes in family members less than 60.
- Family members who have hypertension
- Obesity
- Family history of hyperlipidemia

Prevention

It is quite rare that arteriosclerosis or coronary artery disease requires treatment in someone who is still a child, but the prevention of these diseases should certainly start in the pediatric age group. Medical attention should be directed at identifying children who are high risk for the development of arteriosclerotic disease and the practice of good dietary and exercise habits in the entire population. Known familial hypercholesterolemia requires treatment with diet &/or drugs. Any child who is high risk for the development of coronary artery disease or arteriosclerosis should certainly avoid obesity, cigarette smoking, be monitored for the development of hypertension and have a diet with reduced saturated fats and cholesterol.

Hypertension

Secondary hypertension is much more common than essential hypertension in infants and children. The vast majority of children who have secondary hypertension have it as a result of a renal abnormality (see Chapter 13). The term essential hypertension implies that no known underlying disease is present, and certainly essential hypertension is not a single entity.

Predisposing Conditions
- Family history
- Salt intake (in some individuals)
- Stress
- Obesity

Symptoms

Children with essential hypertension are usually not symptomatic, unless the disease is sustained and then they may have headaches, dizziness, changes in vision, or seizures.

Physical Findings

Blood pressure persistently above the 95th percentile for age on repeated measurements with an appropriate-sized cuff. This is more commonly found in the obese child.

Potential Complications
- Myocardial infarction
- Stroke
- Renal failure

Treatment Plan

Treatment begins with weight reduction, limitation of salt intake, a reasonable exercise program, etc, and may proceed to pharmacologic therapy. The most important management of hypertension for the pediatric population is certainly its prevention. These methods are essentially the same as the prevention of other cardiovascular disease and include a diet low in saturated fats, appropriate body weight for age and size, limited salt intake and a healthy exercise regimen.

Cardiomyopathies

Most primary cardiomyopathies in children are of the dilated type and are usually related to myocarditis, a primary cardiomyopathy, or the use of drugs, particularly Adriamyacin.

Predisposing Conditions
- Family history of primary cardiomyopathies
- Use of drugs associated with the development of cardiomyopathy
- Viral infection (eg, Coxsackie B virus)

Diagnosis

Most patients with cardiomyopathies present in congestive heart failure (see Chapter 17)

Potential Complications

Development of chronic cardiomyopathy, death

Management

Supportive care initially with consideration of heart transplant for those patients who develop chronic cardiomyopathies.

Arrhythmias

AV Block

AV block is uncommon in children. It is divided into first degree block in which the PR interval is prolonged but there is AV conduction, second degree block in which some atrial impulses are not conducted to the ventricles, and third degree block (complete heart block) in which no atrial impulses are conducted to the ventricles. A specific discussion of congenital complete AV block appears below.

Congenital Complete AV Block

Complete heart block can occur in the pediatric population. It is most common as a congenital disease.

Etiology

The majority of congenital complete heart block and the vast majority of pediatric complete heart block are secondary to autoimmune diseases. In these autoimmune diseases the conduction system is damaged by IgG antibodies. Other causes include complex congenital heart disease, abnormal embryonic development of the conduction system, myocarditis, long QT syndrome and prior history of surgical repair of a congenital heart lesion.

Pathophysiology

As described above complete heart block is a situation in which the atria and ventricle function independently with no conduction of atrial impulses to the ventricle.

Predisposing Conditions

Congenital AV block is most commonly seen in infants of mothers with systemic lupus erythematosus; it may also be seen in mothers with rheumatoid arthritis, dermatomyositis or Sjögren syndrome.

Symptoms

• Patients with congenital complete heart block may have ventricular rates lower than 50 beats per minute, may develop evidence of hydrops or may develop heart failure. Some infants with congenital complete heart block do not present at birth but develop heart block within the first three-to-six months of life.

- Older children who have complete heart block are frequently asymptomatic but may have attacks of syncope. Their systolic blood pressure is usually elevated.

Diagnosis

Is suspected clinically and confirmed by electrocardiogram. On electrocardiogram the P-waves and the QRS complexes have no constant relation.

Potential Complication

- Development of congestive heart failure
- Death
- Chronic hypertension and syncope

Management

Depending on the severity of the disease; newborns or older children with complete heart block may require cardiac pacing.

Supraventricular Tachycardia

SVT of Infancy

SVT of infancy is a specific condition in which SVT develops in utero or early in life. It requires emergent management and care. The infant is usually severely ill and in heart failure. Acute treatment with adenosine or cardioversion may be necessary and chronic management with digitalis is usually essential.

NOTE: Remember that in infants verapamil is a contraindicated drug because its use may result in profound hypotension and myocardial depression.

Children are at increased risk of SVT of infancy if they are males or if they have Wolf-Parkinson-White (WPW) syndrome. Most SVT of infancy resolves by one year of age and digitalis is usually discontinued at about that time.

SVT After Infancy

Children or adults may have or develop SVT after infancy if they have an abnormal point of origin of electrical impulses in their atria. Many of these individuals have WPW syndrome. Pharmacologic management is usually attempted in these individuals but episodes of breakthrough SVT with eventual development of congestive failure may occur. Electrical cardiac mapping with catheter ablation of abnormal foci of electrical activity is now frequently done and has been very successful for the correction of this problem.

Jill Stewart

The hematopoietic system includes white blood cells, red blood cells and platelets. This chapter will focus on red blood cell diseases and platelet/coagulation disorders. It is useful to begin with an understanding of the development and production of blood elements, particularly as it impacts various disease states.

Developmental Considerations

Prenatal: Hematopoiesis is the body's system of producing blood cells. The system arises from the mesodermal layer of the embryo and is active at three weeks post conception. By two months of fetal life active hematopoiesis is present primarily in the liver and by six months primary production shifts to the bone marrow. The liver continues its hematopoietic activity until about two weeks after birth. Of note, the spleen, thymus and lymph nodes play a part in hematopoiesis during fetal life as well.

Postnatal: In infants the medullary spaces of most bones contain hematopoietic tissue, but as childhood progresses the marrow in long bones is replaced by fatty tissues. This "yellow" marrow can be recruited to produce blood cells if needed, but primary blood cell production in older children and adults occurs in the ribs, sternum, vertebrae, pelvis, skull, clavicles and scapula.

Red blood cell production requires pluripotential stem cells, erythropoietin stimulation and multiple nutrients, such as iron, folate, vitamin B_{12}, etc. Any abnormality in these three areas can create an over- or (more commonly) under-production of RBCs. Fetal RBCs typically survive 90 days while mature RBCs survive approximately 120 days. All these factors must be considered when evaluating red blood cell disorders.

Hemoglobin is the most important component of RBCs. This oxygen-carrying protein is crucial to tissue metabolism. Hemoglobin is composed of four polypeptide chains bound to two heme groups which reversibly bind O_2. During fetal life Hgb F, $\alpha_2\gamma_2$, predominates (70% at birth) and is gradually replaced by Hgb A, $\alpha_2\beta_2$, predominance (90% by 6-12 months of age). In a normal child the Hgb level is < 2%. Multiple genetic errors in polypeptide production account for the hemoglobinopathies.

RBCs extrude their nucleus during maturation but remain metabolically active, fueled largely by anaerobic glycolysis. Aberrations in these enzyme functions result in electrolyte gradient changes and often changes in RBC shape. These enzymatic abnormalities often manifest as hemolytic anemia.

Platelets are produced from bone marrow megakaryocytes and have a lifespan of 7-10 days. They work in concert with numerous serum proteins in the delicate balance of hemostasis. Any abnormalities in this balance manifest as a coagulation disorder.

Diagnostic Modalities

History

As with all aspects of medicine this component is most important. It should include questions about fatigue, pallor, bleeding, bruising, diet, infections, development, illnesses and family history, particularly of bleeding disorders or gallbladder disease.

Physical Exam

Multiple physical findings may be present with abnormalities of the hematopoietic system. Findings are not exclusive to hematologic abnormalities but may give important clues for diagnosis.

Vitals

tachycardia - anemia

tachypnea - anemia causing CHF

Skin

pallor, pale palmar creases - anemia

jaundice - hemolysis

petechiae - thrombocytopenia

plethora - polycythemia

bruises/purpura - coagulopathy

HEENT

scleral icterus - hemolysis

pale conjunctiva - anemia

maxillary hyperplasia - hemoglobinopathy

epistaxis - coagulopathy

gingival hemorrhage - coagulopathy

glossitis - B_{12} deficiency

CV

systolic murmur - anemia

Abdomen

splenomegaly - sequestration of abnormal cells

Extremities

koilonychia (spooning of fingernails) - iron deficiency

Laboratory

Numerous laboratory tests, as indicated by the history and exam, are utilized in diagnosis:

CBC

The complete blood count provides much useful information

Hgb - hemoglobin concentration

Hct - % of concentration of RBCs in blood

RBC - red blood cell count

RBC Indexes

MCV - (Mean Corpuscular Volume) - average volume of red cell

MCH - (Mean Corpuscular Hemoglobin) - weight of Hgb in average red cell

MCHC - (Mean Corpuscular Hemoglobin Concentration) - average concentration of Hgb in a given volume of packed red blood cells. (An increase suggests spherocytosis.)

RDW - (Red cell Distribution Width) - Measure of heterogeneity of RBC sizes

Platelet count

Reticulocyte Count - nucleated RBCs. Normal 1-2%. May be higher in hemorrhage or hemolysis.

Peripheral Smear - Manual observation gives invaluable information regarding morphology and color of cells.

anisocytosis - varied sizes

poikilocytosis - varied shapes

acanthocytes - spiculated cells

hypochromia - pale appearance of cells

Iron Studies -

serum iron

serum ferritin -reflection of iron storage in tissues

total iron binding capacity (TIBC)

% saturation of TIBC

Free Erythrocyte Porphyrins (FEP) - heme precursor

Erythrocyte Osmotic Fragility Test - increased fragility of incubated RBCs is suggestive of hereditary spherocytosis.

Hemoglobin Electrophoresis - quantitative determination of hemoglobin variants

Bone Marrow Aspirate and Biopsy - typically obtained from posterior iliac crest which allows assessment of cellularity, distribution and maturation of cells including abnormal cells.

PT - Assessment of Factors II, V, VII and X

PTT - Assessment of Factors VIII, IX, XI and XII

Mixing Study - Normal plasma is added to patients plasma. If repeat PTT normalizes then a deficiency state is present.

Bleeding Time - Assessment of vascular and platelet function. Normal 4-8 minutes.

Anemias can be diagnostically quite complex.   The following chart is a useful guide for interpreting laboratory data:

RBC Morphology and Indexes

Microcytic-hypochromic anemia

    Free Erythrocyte Protoporphyrin

    Low free erythrocyte protoporphyrin (FEP)

        Thalassemia

    High free erythrocyte protoporphyrin (FEP)

        Serum Ferritin

        High/normal ferritin

            Lead poisoning

            Chronic disease

            Pyridoxine deficiency

            Sideroblastic anemia

        Low ferritin

            Iron deficiency

Macrocytic-normochromic

    Megaloblastic anemia (folate, B_{12} deficiency)

    Aplastic/hypoplastic anemia

    Fanconi's anemia

    Hypothyroidism

    Congenital dyserythropoietic anemia

    Hepatic disease

Normocytic-normochromic anemia

    Reticulocyte Count

    Low reticulocyte count

        Platelet Count

        Low platelet count

            Bone Marrow Examination

            Bone marrow: Blasts present

                Leukemia

                Metastatic tumor

            Bone marrow: Blasts absent

                Aplastic/hypoplastic anemia

                Lipid storage disease

        High/normal platelet count

            Renal disease

            Infection

            Inflammation

Chronic disease
Hypothyroidism
Diamond-Blackfan anemia
Transient erythroblastopenia
Congenital dyserthropoetic anemia
Protein malnutrition
High reticulocyte count
Indirect Bilirubin
Normal indirect bilirubin
blood loss
Elevated indirect bilirubin
Coombs' Test
Positive Coombs' test
Autoimmune hemolytic anemia
Isoimmune hemolytic anemia (Rh, ABO)
Incompatible transfusion
Negative Coombs' test
Fragmented Cells on Peripheral Smear
Burr, helmet cells/schistocytes present
Hemolytic Uremic syndrome
DIC
Burr, helmet cells/schistocytes absent
Osmotic Fragility Test
RBC fragility test abnormal
Spherocytosis
Stomatocytosis
Elliptocytosis
Vitamin E deficiency
RBC fragility normal
Hemoglobin Electrophoresis
Hgb electrophoresis abnormal
Sickle cell disease
Hgb SC disease
Hgb S-beta-thalassemia
Hgb electrophoresis normal
G6PD deficiency
Pyruvate kinase deficiency
Elliptocytosis
Stomatocytosis

CHAPTER 11

Disease Profiles

This section provides an overview of many diseases - these include:
    Pancytopenias
        Fanconi syndrome
        Acquired
    Anemias
        Decreased Production
            Inadequate Precursors
                Diamond-Blackfan
                Transient Erythroblastopenia of Childhood
                Acquired
            Inadequate Production Despite Normal Precursors
                Chronic Disease
                Physiologic Anemia
            Inadequate Synthetic Factors
                Folate
                B_{12}
                Ortoic acidurig
                Iron deficiency
                Sideroblastic anemia
                Lead poisoning
        Increased Destruction
            Structural Defects
                Hereditary Spherocytosis
                Hereditary Elliptocytosis
                PNH
                Stomatocytosis
            Enzymatic Defects
                Pyruvate Kinase Deficiency
                G6PD Deficiency
            Immune Mediated
                Hemolytic Disease of the Newborn
                Autoimmune Hemolytic Anemia
    Coagulation Disorders
        Abnormalities of Platelets
            Inherited Thrombocytopenias
                Wiskott-Aldrich Syndrome
                TAR Syndrome
                Kasabach-Merritt Syndrome

Abnormalities of Protein Factors
    Factor VIII Deficiency
    Factor IX Deficiency
    Von Willebrand Disease
    Vitamin K Defficiency
    Disseminated Intravascular Coagulation
Hemoglobinopathies
    Sickle Cell Anemia
    Sickle Cell Trait
    Hemoglobin C Disorders
    Beta-thalassemias
    Alpha-thalassemias
Polycythemias
    Erythrocytosis
    Polycythemia Rubra Vera
Coagulation Disorders

Pancytopenias

Aplasia of the bone marrow or acquired damage to its hematopoietic elements results in profound depression of all the formed elements of blood. Clinically the consequences of thrombocytopenia and neutropenia are most striking, but anemia occurs as well.

Constitutional Aplastic Pancytopenia (Fanconi syndrome)

Pathogenesis

Autosomal recessive disorder with variable penetrance associated with chromosomal fragility in all cells of the body, including the hematopoietic system.

Clinical Features

2/3 of affected patients have associated anomalies such as absence of radii and thumbs, short stature, hyperpigmentation of the skin or cardiac and renal abnormalities. Onset of pancytopenia occurs on average at 6-8 years of age.

Laboratory Findings

Severe pancytopenia
Macrocytic RBCs
Bone marrow hypocellularity
Increase of Hgb F to 5-15%
10-70% abnormal chromosome configurations (normally changes
    seen in < 10%).

Treatment

Bone marrow transplantation is definitive therapy; however, many patients exhibit improvement with androgenic steroids. Supportive care with platelet/RBC transfusions and antibiotics is also critical.

Acquired Pancytopenia

Pathogenesis

Multiple etiologies have been documented including

Replacement of normal marrow by other tissue (eg, neuroblastoma, ALL)

Infectious agents (eg, parvovirus, hepatitis)

Antibiotic exposure (eg, chloramphenicol, sulfonamides)

Chemical exposure (eg, benzene)

Malignancy therapy (eg, methotrexate, 6-MP; ionizing radiation)

In about 50% of cases no etiologic agent is identified and is therefore termed idiopathic.

Clinical Features

May have features of underlying malignancy if present, but typically presents with hemorrhage secondary to thrombocytopenia. Symptoms of anemia and infection become apparent later.

Laboratory Findings

Severe pancytopenia

Normal chromosome configuration

Treatment

Bone marrow transplantation is the treatment of choice. Some success with immunotherapy (eg, anti-thymocyte globulin, dexamethasone, cyclosporin) has been reported. Supportive care with platelet/RBC transfusions and antibiotics is usually necessary. Unfortunately about 2/3 of patients die within six months of diagnosis.

Anemias

Anemia is defined as the reduction of the hemoglobin or hematocrit below two standard deviations of the mean. It is important to recognize that normal values vary with age. As a general rule, physiologic disturbances are minor until hemoglobin falls below 7-8 g/dL. Manifestations such as pallor and fatigue may be subtle if the onset of anemia is gradual. However, symptoms may progress to cardiac dilatation and congestive heart failure if not treated appropriately. Physiologic adjustments to anemia include tachycardia, increased cardiac output and a shift of the oxygen-dissociation curve to the right, providing more efficient transfer of oxygen to the tissues.

It is important to remember that anemia is not a disease itself but a symptom of an underlying problem. Clinically anemias are classified according to morphologic appearance of the RBC and mean corpuscular volume (eg, hypochromic microcytic; macrocytic; normochromic normocytic) as shown in the previous chart. For purposes of this overview anemias will be categorized into two large groups based on etiologies:

- Decreased Production of Red Blood Cells
- Increased Destruction of Red Blood Cells

Decreased Production of Red Blood Cells
Inadequate Precursors
Congenital Pure Red Blood Cell Anemia (Diamond-Blackfan syndrome)
Pathogenesis
Isolated deficiency of RBC precursors in bone marrow with a presumed genetic basis suggested by familial occurrences.

Clinical Features
About half of affected infants appear pale in the first week of life and profound anemia is evident by 2-6 mo. of age. Occasionally associated with phenotypic abnormalities such as triphalangeal thumbs and Turner syndrome.

Laboratory Findings
Macrocytic, normochromic anemia
Low reticulocyte count
Increased serum erythropoietin
Increased Hgb F
Increased serum iron
Decreased TIBC
Bone marrow - markedly reduced RBC precursors

Treatment
Over half of patients respond to corticosteroid therapy. Those who do not respond may require blood transfusions at 4-8 week intervals. Long-term complications from corticosteroid therapy and hemosiderosis secondary to multiple RBC transfusions are quite problematic. These complications include growth retardation, delayed puberty, diabetes mellitus, hepatosplenomegaly and secondary thrombocytopenia, congestive heart failure and often death.

Aggressive iron chelation therapy and attempts at corticosteroid weaning optimize care. Spontaneous remission may occur.

Transient Erythroblastopenia of Childhood (TEC)
Pathogenesis
> This severe reversible anemia is of unknown etiology but likely has an autoimmune basis with serum inhibitors directed at erythroid stem cells.

Clinical Features
> Slow insidious development of anemia in previously normal children 6 mo - 5 yr of age.

Laboratory Findings
> Normochromic normocytic anemia
> Decreased reticulocytes
> Increased serum iron and iron saturation
> Normal Hgb F

Treatment
> Transfusions may be necessary with severe anemia causing cardiac decompensation. However, typically no treatment is required and spontaneous recovery occurs in 2 - 4 weeks.

Acquired Pure Red Cell Anemias
Pathogenesis
> Multiple etiologies can create isolated reduced red blood cell precursors including erythropoietin inhibiting antibodies, erythroblast antibodies, inhibitors of heme synthesis, viral infections and an ill-defined association with thymomas.

Clinical Features
> Dependent on etiology but typically have slow onset of anemia. If patient also has an underlying hemolytic anemia causing decreased mature RBC survival time, one may experience a dramatic aplastic crisis.

Laboratory Findings
> Normochromic, normocytic anemia
> Decreased reticulocytes
> Increased serum iron
> Bone marrow - reduction in RBC precursors

Treatment
> Dependent on etiology. May require supportive RBC transfusions, resection of thymoma or immunosuppressive medications. Prognosis is also dependent on etiology with spontaneous recovery in two weeks if secondary to viral infections.

Inadequate Production Despite Normal Precursors
Anemia of Chronic Disease
Pathogenesis

Occurs as a complication of chronic systemic diseases associated with infection, inflammation or tissue breakdown. RBC life span is moderately decreased secondary to increased RBC destruction by the reticuloendothelial system. More important is the relative failure of the bone marrow response reflecting both hypoactive marrow and inadequate erythropoietin production. Additionally, abnormalities of iron metabolism may worsen anemia.

Clinical Features

Few symptoms of the mild-moderate anemia occur with the important features attributable to the underlying disease (eg, SLE; JRA; renal diseases; osteomyelitis; ulcerative colitis).

Laboratory Findings

Normochromic, normocytic anemia (Hgb 6-9 g/dL)
    occasionally hypochromic microcytic secondary to
    abnormal iron metabolism
Decreased or normal reticulocyte count
Increased FEP
Decreased serum iron
Increased ferritin (acute phase reactant)
Normal TIBC

Treatment

Management of underlying disease

Physiologic Anemia of Infancy
Pathogenesis

"Anemia" is a misnomor as events leading to low Hgb are normal physiologic adaptations to extra-uterine life. Term infants experience a drop in hemoglobin to about 9 g/dL at 6-8 weeks of age. Multiple adaptations create this effect. Newborns are relatively polycythemic secondary to erythropoetin stimulation from low intrauterine oxygen levels. At birth p_aO_2 levels dramatically increase and erythropoietin production ceases. Decreased hematopoesis therefore contributes to "anemia" with erythropoetin production restimulated as Hgb falls. Other contributing factors are the relatively short life span of fetal blood cells and the dramatic increase in blood volume during the first 2 months of life.

Clinical Features

Asymptomatic unless other processes aggravating anemia are present such as blood loss, hemolysis or nutritional deficits.

Laboratory Findings

Hgb 9-11 g/dL

Treatment

None required. Nutritional counseling should be provided as needed.

Inadequate Synthetic Factors
Folic Acid Deficiency
Pathogenesis

Folic acid deficiency impairs DNA synthesis. RNA synthesis is less affected allowing cytoplasmic maturation to progress which accounts for the macrocytic appearance of RBCs. Folic acid deficiency can arise for multiple reasons.

- inadequate intake - infants fed goat's milk require folic acid supplementation
- increased demand - folic acid requirements increase dramatically with pregnancy, malignancies and chronic hemolysis
- impaired absorption - chronic enteritis (eg, Crohn's Disease, Celiac Disease) may impair small intestine absorption of dietary folate
- abnormal metabolism - drugs such as trimethoprim - sulfamethoxazole, pyrimethamine, phenytoin, methotrexate and oral contraceptives all can impact folate metabolism causing megaloblastic anemia.

Clinical Features

Anemia appears 3-6 mo after onset of deficiency. May manifest with FTT, irritability, chronic diarrhea.

Laboratory Findings

Macrocytic anemia
Hypersegmented neutrophil nuclei

Serum folic acid level 3 ng/ml (normal 5-20 ng/ml)
RBC folate level < 150 ng/ml (normal 150-600 ng/ml)
Increased LDH

Treatment

Dependent on etiology. Folic acid supplementation produces a hematologic response within 72 hours. Transfusions are rarely required.

Vitamin B_{12} Deficiency

Pathogenesis

B_{12} deficiency impacts DNA synthesis, leading to a macrocytic anemia. Deficiency occurs with inadequate intake or abnormal absorption. Dietary deficiency is rare but can occur in the breast fed infant of a strict vegetarian. Absorption problems are much more common given the complex nature of B_{12} metabolism. B_{12} must bind with intrinsic factor, produced by gastric parietal cells. This complex then must reach the terminal ileum, where calcium is required for its site-specific absorption. Transcobalamin is then necessary to transport B_{12} in the plasma. Abnormalities in this sequence can create a deficiency. Examples:

- Absence of Intrinsic Factor - juvenile pernicious anemia
- Gastric mucosal atrophy/Achlorhydria
- Abnormal terminal ileum - regional enteritis, tuberculosis
- Absent terminal ileum - surgical resection secondary to necrotizing enterocolitis or Crohn's Disease
- Competition for vitamin - bacterial overgrowth; tapeworm *Diphyllobothrium latum* infestation
- Intestinal absorption defect - A familial syndrome of cutaneous candidiasis, hypoparathyroidism and other endocrine deficiencies can be associated with B_{12} absorption defect. When an absorption defect is associated with proteinuria it is known as Imerslund syndrome.

Clinical Features

Onset at 9 months - 10 years of age as body stores are depleted. May present with diarrhea, irritability, anorexia, listlessness and neurologic manifestations such as ataxia, paresthesias, hyperreflexia, clonus and Babinski signs. On physical exam a classic finding is a smooth, red, painful tongue.

Laboratory Findings

Macrocytic anemia

Hypersegmented neutrophil nuclei

Serum B_{12} level <100 pg/ml

Elevated LDH

Increased urinary excretion of methylmalonic acid

Schilling Test - utilized to evaluate B_{12} absorption. Radioactive labelled B_{12} is ingested. In a normal person this binds to intrinsic factor and is absorbed in the terminal ileum. As a consequence of its protein binding none is normally excreted in the urine. A large nonradioactive "flushing" dose of B_{12} is then administered parenterally. This causes 10-30% of the previous radioactive dose to be excreted in the urine. Less than this implies an absorption defect which can be further evaluated by administering intrinsic factor with the radioactive B_{12}. If excretion after a flushing dose normalizes, then a diagnosis of pernicious anemia can be made. If excretion remains low an intestinal defect is implicated.

Treatment

B_{12} supplementation is definitive therapy with maintenance doses of 1mg IM monthly. If neurologic involvement presents 1 mg IM daily for two weeks is necessary. If transcobalamin deficiency is present massive parenteral doses of B_{12} are required.

Orotic Aciduria
Pathogenesis
Autosomal recessive deficiency of orotate phosphoribosyl transferase or orotidine -5-phosphate decarboxylase. These enzymes are essential in the production of pyrimidines without which DNA and RNA synthesis is impaired. Abnormality is present in all cells but most dramatic in the hematopoietic system.

Clinical Features
Failure to thrive and developmental delay are frequently noted along with symptoms of anemia.

Laboratory Findings
Macrocytic anemia

Neutropenia

Orotic acid crystals in urine

Treatment
Administration of pyrimidine precursors found beyond the metabolic pathway block normalizes RBC production.

Iron Deficiency
Pathogenesis
Iron is necessary for hemoglobin synthesis and in its absence a dramatic anemia can ensue. Deficiency can occur with blood loss or insufficient dietary intake. Blood loss can occur at any age and for any reason but commonly occurs during infancy from the GI tract secondary to cow's milk protein intolerance. Dietary insufficiency often occurs in infancy if milk or cereals without iron fortification are ingested. This propensity for infants to develop a deficiency is related to the precarious balance of iron metabolism in the first months of life. In the normal newborn iron stores, including iron reclaimed from the high neonatal Hgb concentrations, are sufficient for blood formation for 6-9 months. Thereafter, a diet of 8-15 mg/day of iron is required as only 10% of ingested iron is absorbed. If an infant's body store of iron is low (secondary to prematurity; pre or perinatal hemorrhage) or if iron-fortified foods are not offered a child is quite likely to develop this, **the most common of all anemias**.

Clinical Features

Commonly presents at 6-24 months of age as a consequence of dietary inadequacy. Can present earlier if iron stores depleted as a consequence of other factors. Often insidious presentation with pallor the most important clue. Irritability and anorexia present in severe cases.

Laboratory Findings

Hypochromic microcytic anemia
Decreased serum Ferritin (<10 ng/ml)
Decreased serum iron (<30 mcg/dL)
Increased TIBC (>350 mcg/dL)
Decreased % saturation TIBC (<15%)
Increased FEP (>50 mcg/dL)
Normal or slightly increased reticulocyte count
Guaiac positive stool (1/3 of cases)

Treatment

Oral administration of elemental iron 6 mg/kg/day in three divided doses produces a responsive reticulocytosis within 72 hours. Fe replacement should be continued at least 6 weeks after RBC count has normalized in order to replace body stores. Equally important is attention to the underlying etiology, including an evaluation for blood loss &/or dietary counseling.

Sideroblastic Anemia

Pathogenesis

Ill-defined abnormalities in iron or heme metabolism inhibit hemoglobin synthesis creating anemia. Iron accumulates in mitochondria of erythroid precursors creating the typical appearance of red blood cells with a perinuclear collar of hemosiderin granules termed a ringed sideroblast. Can be X-linked recessive or acquired.

Clinical Features

Inherited trait is symptomatic by late childhood and splenomegaly is a common finding. The acquired disorder presents in alcoholics or adults with inflammatory or malignant processes.

Laboratory Findings

Hypochromic microcytic anemia

Increased serum iron

Normal or increased FEP

Peripheral smear - RBC stippling

Bone marrow - ringed sideroblasts

Treatment

Some cases are responsive to pyridoxine (β_6) therapy in doses of 200-500 mg/day. Of note, no other findings of pyridoxine deficiency are observed in these patients.

Lead Poisoning

Pathogenesis

Environmental exposure to lead can be toxic to the CNS, renal and hematopoietic systems. Severity of toxicity is directly related to the level of lead absorption. The hematopoietic system is affected by lead's inhibition of two enzymes (ferrochelatase and porphobilinogen) necessary in the pathway of heme synthesis. This inhibition creates elevations of δ-aminolevulinic acid and FEP along the metabolic pathway, which are utilized in diagnosis. The most significant source of environmental lead is household dust and dirt, as substantial reductions of lead in food, air and drinking water have been mandated.

Clinical Features

Symptoms are generally nonspecific but occur most frequently in toddlers. Neurologic manifestations such as seizures, behavior problems, mental retardation, irritability and acute encephalopathy are possible. In addition recurrent episodes of vomiting, abdominal pain and constipation herald GI involvement.

Laboratory Findings

Hypochromic microcytic anemia

Venous lead level > 10 mcg/dL

Increased FEP

Increased plasma and urine δ-aminolevulinic acid

Increased reticulocytes

Peripheral smear - basophilic stippling

CSF: pleocytosis, increased protein and pressure in cases of toxic encephalopathy

Treatment

Chelation therapy is indicated for children with significantly elevated lead levels. The exact level warranting medical intervention is controversial but generally ≥ 25 mcg/dL. Agents such as CaEDTA, DMSA and BAL can be utilized. Close followup is mandatory as serum lead levels can rebound into the toxic range as chronic lead deposited in the bones is leached into the soft tissues after treatment. Equally important is environmental control. A complete evaluation of the child's environment is required in order to eliminate additional exposure.

Increased Destruction of Red Blood Cells
Structural Defects
Hereditary Spherocytosis
Pathogenesis

Autosomal dominant condition with 25% of cases sporadic new mutations. The defect involves spectrin, which is a structural protein crucial in maintaining the RBC shape. Without this protein support structure the cell loses its biconcave disc shape and becomes spherical. The spherical shape makes the RBC less deformable when passing through small vasculature and consequently is often trapped in the splenic sinusoids. In addition, the RBC membrane is excessively permeable to sodium. This creates a metabolic crisis as more ATP is needed to drive the cation pump and maintain the normal electrical gradient. The spleen is a metabolically stressful environment for these RBCs, as the glucose and oxygen concentrations necessary for ATP production are relatively low. These two RBC defects create a chronic hemolytic process in the spleen.

Clinical Features

Presentation varies with age. Newborns often have severe anemia and jaundice. Older children present with pallor and splenomegaly. Adolescents often present with pigmented gallstone cholecystitis secondary to chronic hemolysis. Occasionally in the face of a superseding viral infection (eg, parvovirus) patients may present with aplastic crisis as the bone marrow is unable to maintain its accelerated replenishment of destroyed RBCs.

Laboratory Findings

Normochromic, normocytic anemia
Peripheral smear - spherocytes
Elevated MCHC
Increased reticulocytes (5-20%)
Unconjugated hyperbilirubinemia
Positive RBS Osmotic Fragility Test

Treatment

Supportive care with transfusions as needed and careful attention to increased bone marrow nutrient needs such as folate and iron. Splenectomy is the definitive treatment but usually is deferred until age 6 years. Splenectomy reduces RBC destruction and the associated complications but RBC spherocytes remain. Pneumococcal vaccination to allow immune system development prior to splenectomy is standard of care.

Hereditary Elliptocytosis

Pathogenesis

Autosomal dominant condition with abnormal spectrin dimer interactions creating elliptical-shaped RBCs. Generally benign except when spherocytes are also present creating a moderate chronic hemolysis. Elliptocytosis gene is linked with the Rh locus.

Clinical Features

Variable clinical course with only about 10% of patients experiencing ongoing hemolysis. Features such as neonatal jaundice, splenomegaly, cholelithiasis, and medullary expansion of bones may be present.

Laboratory Findings

Normochromic, normocytic anemia
Peripheral smear - elliptocytes, poikilocytes
Increased reticulocyte count
Unconjugated hyperbilirubinemia

Treatment

Asymptomatic patients require no intervention; however, those with ongoing hemolysis benefit from pneumococcal immunization followed by splenectomy at 6 years of age.

Paroxysmal Nocturnal Hemoglobinuria

Pathogenesis

Ill-defined inciting etiology but mechanism is related to an acquired deficiency of decay-accelerating factor. This factor normally is present in the RBC membrane. In its absence the alternative complement pathway is triggered by C3b causing intravascular hemolysis. Episodes of hemolysis often occur at night, presumably when serum pCO_2 rises and pH falls. Chronic leukopenia and thrombocytopenia may be present as well as aplastic pancytopenia.

Clinical Features

Nocturnal and morning hemoglobinuria is the classic feature often accompanied by abdominal, back and head pain. Serious complications such as thrombosis, thromboembolic phenomenon or pyogenic infections may also be initial manifestations.

Laboratory Findings

Nocturnal hemoglobinuria
Positive Ham test - Increased lysis in acidified serum
Positive sucrose lysis test - increased lysis in isotonic
low ionic strength solutions.
Decreased decay-accelerating factor
Decreased RBC acetylcholinesterase activity

Treatment

Supportive care with transfusions as needed. Iron supplementation is often needed due to its excessive loss in the urine. Patients with thromboses may benefit from anticoagulation therapy. Splenectomy is not useful as the hemolysis is intravascular, but bone marrow transplantation has been utilized with some success.

Stomatocytosis
Pathogenesis
Rare hereditary condition with extreme RBC membrane permeability to cations (eg, sodium) and resulting hemolytic anemia. Similar abnormality may be acquired with other conditions such as liver disease.

Clinical Features
Generally mild symptoms but occasionally can have severe hemolysis and subsequent anemia and jaundice.

Laboratory Findings
Peripheral smear - swollen cup-shaped RBCs with central slit or stoma

Treatment
Splenectomy may be palliative but not curative in the patient with severe hemolysis.

Enzymatic Defects
Pyruvate Kinase Deficiency
Pathogenesis
Autosomal recessive decrease in RBC pyruvate kinase content or activity. This enzyme catalyzes the final step in the glycolytic pathway leading to eventual ATP production. In this deficiency ATP production is inadequate to operate the cation pump essential to maintain normal cellular Na+ and K+ balance. Intracellular K+ is lost and Na+ accumulates. As a result the RBC lifespan is markedly reduced.

Clinical Features
Variable presentations ranging from severe neonatal hemolysis with anemia, jaundice and even kernicterus to a mild well-compensated hemolysis noted first in adulthood. Pallor and splenomegaly are usually present. The midwestern Amish have a high incidence of severe hemolytic disease.

Laboratory Findings
Decreased RBC pyruvate kinase activity
Increased reticulocyte count
Peripheral smear - macrocytosis (secondary to reticulocytes)
Unconjugated hyperbilirubinemia

Treatment

Supportive care with RBC transfusions as needed. Recurrent hemolytic episodes may require splenectomy after age 6 years. Of note, the reticulocyte count often paradoxically increases further after splenectomy due to their prolonged survival in the circulation.

Glucose-6-Phosphate Dehydrogenase (G6PD) Deficiency
Pathogenesis

G6PD is an enzyme of the pentose phosphate pathway. This pathway functions to produce NADPH which is necessary in the conversion of oxidized to reduced glutathione. Reduced glutathione is essential for the inactivation of any oxidant compound in the RBC. Oxidant compounds can cause heme and globin chains to dissociate by oxidation of sulfhydryl groups. The denatured globin can then precipitate as a Heinz body which in turn damages the RBC membrane. A deficiency of G6PD thus leads to accelerated splenic removal and also intravascular lysis of RBCs. This deficiency is x-linked recessive with over 100 variants identified. The normal enzyme is designated G6PD B+ with two primary variants identified as G6PD A- found in black and G6PD B- found in Mediterranean and Oriental ethnic groups.

Clinical Features

Typically, patients present with a drug-induced episodic hemolytic anemia. Common inciting drugs are sulfonamides, antipyretics, napthaquinolones and antimalarials such as primaquine. Other oxidative agents may also trigger the hemolysis, such as infection or ingestion of fava beans, a Mediterranean dietary staple. The degree of hemolysis varies with the inciting agent, the amount ingested and the severity of the enzyme deficiency. Most will present 48-72 hours after exposure but the B-variant will experience a more severe course while the A-variant will commonly have self-limited hemolysis. Presentation can also occur with neonatal hyperbilirubinemia despite no known exposures.

Laboratory Findings
Normochromic, normocytic anemia
Peripheral smear - Heinz bodies
Hemoglobinuria
Unconjugated hyperbilirubinemia
G6PD activity ≤ 10% of normal

Treatment
Spontaneous recovery occurs but supportive transfusions are sometimes needed. Identification of patients with this common deficiency and prevention of oxidant exposures is optimal management.

Immune Mediated
Hemolytic Disease of Newborn
Pathogenesis
Hemolysis occurs with transplacental passage of maternal antibody active against red blood cell antigens of the infant. The D antigen of the Rh group and ABO blood type antigens are most frequently involved. Rh incompatibility arises when a Rh- mother is exposed to an Rh+ infant. A brisk maternal IgG response ensues after only 1 ml of Rh+ blood exposure. This IgG in turn crosses the placenta and may cause catastrophic in utero hemolysis and hydrops fetalis. ABO incompatibility typically occurs when a B+ or more commonly A+ infant is born to an O+ mother. Maternal anti-A or anti-B antibody creates mild-moderate hemolysis in the infant. These antibodies are usually IgM and, therefore, cannot cross the placenta but may be present in small IgG fractions which explains the milder clinical course.

Clinical Features
Infants with Rh incompatibility typically have severe hemolysis and subsequent multiple organ system dysfunction including the cardiac, pulmonary and hepatic systems. The severity of involvement is dependent on the immune response by the mother. Infants with ABO incompatibility generally develop jaundice in the first 24 hours of life but rarely experience significant complications.

Laboratory Findings

Normochromic, normocytic anemia

Maternal - Infant blood antigen incompatibility (Rh or ABO)

Coombs' positive

Unconjugated hyperbilirubinemia

Increased reticulocytes

Treatment

Infants with ABO incompatibility require management of hyperbilirubinemia with phototherapy and, rarely, exchange transfusions. Infants with Rh disease require intensive multi-system support including management of hyperbilirubinemia. Due to its devastating effects Rh disease is best managed by prevention. Administration of RhoGAM (anti-D globulin) at 28 weeks gestation and again at birth to Rh- mothers is very effective.

Autoimmune Hemolytic Anemia

Pathogenesis

Abnormal IgG or IgM antibodies directed against red blood cells are produced by the patient. IgG antibodies are known as warm-reactive in that they are maximally reactive at 37° C. They coat RBCs but do not activate the complement cascade so RBCs are consequently destroyed by the reticuloendothelial system. IgM antibodies are known as cold-reactive in that they are maximally reactive at colder temperatures. They can activate the complement system so hemolysis occurs intravascularly. The abnormal production of these antibodies is incompletely understood, but often accompanies viral infections, drug exposure, lymphomas or autoimmune disorders such as SLE in the case of IgG. Abnormal IgM antibodies often accompany Mycoplasma and Epstein-Barr virus infections.

Clinical Features

Vary according to associated disease. Children with viral infections experience acute illness with pallor, fever, jaundice, hemoglobinuria, and splenomegaly. Patients with autoimmune disorders may experience a prolonged chronic hemolysis.

Laboratory Findings

Normochromic, normocytic anemia

Coombs' positive

Unconjugated hyperbilirubinemia

Increased reticulocytes

Positive IgM cold agglutination

Treatment

Supportive care and transfusions as needed. Some patients will respond to immunosuppressive doses of prednisone 2.5-6 mg/kg/day which can be slowly tapered. Most cases are self-limited but some require splenectomy and additional immunosuppressive therapies.

Hemoglobinopathies

Structural abnormalities of hemoglobin as a result of molecular defects in globin-gene DNA are classified as hemoglobinopathies. These defects can effect single amino acids in the polypeptide structure or delete an entire globin gene. Two distinct defects can be found in the same person.

Sickle Cell Anemia (Homozygous Hgb S)

Pathogenesis

Homozygous defect on chromosome 11 encoding for a valine substitution for glutamic acid at the 6th position of β chains. When this hemoglobin is deoxygenated a solubility problem arises as molecular polymers can form and aggregate into rigid crystal-like rods. This in turn distorts the RBC into a sickle shape. These sickled RBCs are subsequently destroyed prematurely causing anemia. In addition their unusual shape leads to microvasculature sludging and possible obstruction. Tissue infarction follows and can occur in any organ.

Clinical Features

Newborns are asymptomatic as they have a preponderance of Hgb F. As Hgb F levels fall and abnormal Hgb S levels rise symptoms occur at 4-6 months of age. Avascular necrosis in the small bones of the hand and foot causing painful swelling called dactylitis is often the first manifestation. Acute painful episodes termed vaso-occlusive crises with head, chest, back, abdominal and extremity pain become a chronic recurrent event. They occur when hypoxia, acidosis or infection creates increased sickling. Complications such as cerebrovascular strokes, pulmonary infarctions, splenic sequestration, renal concentrating defects, priapism, aplastic anemia and overwhelming sepsis with encapsulated bacteria secondary to splenic dysfunction can occur. Disease commonly involves the black population.

Laboratory Findings

Normochromic, normocytic anemia

Increased reticulocytes

Unconjugated hyperbilirubinemia

Peripheral smear - sickled cells, poikilocytes

Hgb electrophoresis -　　　　Hgb S 80-95%

　　　　　　　　　　　　　　Hgb F 2-20%

Treatment

Management is directed toward prevention of the multiple complications. Daily antibiotic prophylaxis, complete immunizations including pneumococcal vaccination and parental education about the potential seriousness of fever are important in minimizing morbidity and mortality. Febrile patients should be examined, blood cultures obtained and IV/IM antibiotics administered until sepsis is ruled out. Vaso-occlusive episode prevention involves avoidance of dehydration, hypoxia, acidosis. Treatment includes hydration, analgesics and occasionally RBC transfusions.

Sickle Cell Trait (Heterozygous Hgb S)

Pathogenesis

Heterozygous expression of abnormal sickle hemoglobin encoded on chromosome 11. Normal Hgb A is also expressed so sickling occurs only with significant hypoxic stress. RBCs exhibit resistance to malarial parasite invasion and consequently this gene is frequently found in areas endemic for *Plasmodium falciparum* malaria.

Clinical Manifestations

Generally asymptomatic; however, vaso-occlusive events may occur with severe hypoxia. Adolescents often will have urinary frequency secondary to a renal concentrating defect or painless hematuria. About 10% of USA blacks are affected.

Laboratory Findings

Normal hematologic valves

Hgb electrophoresis　Hgb A 52-65%

　　　　　　　　　　　Hgb S 32-45%

Treatment

No intervention is required unless rare vaso-occlusive events occur.

Hemoglobin C Disorders (Hgb CC; Hgb AC; Hgb SC)

Pathogenesis

Abnormal β-globin gene on chromosome 11 encoding for a lysine substitution for glutamic acid at the 6th position. Pathophysiology is dependent on degree of expression and presence of any other abnormal globin genes. In the homozygous state (Hgb CC) moderate hemolysis occurs in the reticuloendothelial system. In the heterozygous state (Hgb AC) no symptoms are identified. When Hgb S is expressed along with Hgb C (Hgb SC) a sequence of events similar to sickle cell disease occurs. Hgb C participates in the molecular polymerization of deoxygenated Hgb S creating rigid rods which effectively sickle RBCs; consequently, the process of vaso-occlusion occurs.

Clinical Manifestation

Variable. Hgb CC disease is present in 1 in 10,000 USA blacks and manifests with signs of moderate hemolytic anemia and splenomegaly. Hgb AC disease is present in 3% of USA blacks and is asymptomatic. Hgb SC manifests with painful episodes and other vaso-occlusive symptoms much like sickle cell disease although the clinical course is usually not as severe. Bone infarctions are frequent complications.

Laboratory Findings

Hgb CC	normochromic, normocytic anemia
	increased reticulocytes
	peripheral smear - target cells, spherocytes
Hgb AC	normal hematologic parameters
	peripheral smear - target cells
Hgb SC	normochromic, normocytic anemia
	increased reticulocytes
	peripheral smear - sickled cells, target cells
Hgb electrophoresis	Hgb S 45-50%
	Hgb C 45-50%
	Hgb F 2-5%

Treatment

Supportive care is given as needed. The management of Hgb SC disease is identical to that of sickle cell anemia.

Beta-thalassemias

Pathogenesis

Abnormalities in transcription of mRNA from the β-globin genes on chromosome 11 are the most common causes of β-thalassemias. A β° mutation denotes complete absence of production and a β^+ mutation denotes decreased production of β chains. These mutations can occur on both chromosomes (homozygous); on one chromosome (heterozygous) or in combination with other globin chain abnormalities. When β chains are deficient normal Hgb A cannot be produced leading to compensatory increases in Hgb F and Hgb A_2. When the compensatory mechanism is overwhelmed varying stages of anemia can result. Excess α chains precipitate in RBCs as α_4 tetramers and contribute to anemia due to hemolysis.

Clinical Features

Dependent on genetic abnormality. Often found in African or Mediterranean descendants as abnormality protective against *Plasmodium falciparum* malaria.

β°/β° - Cooley Anemia is complete absence of β-chain production. These children present at 6-12 mo. with severe progressive anemia and hepatosplenomegaly. Compensatory extramedullary hematopoiesis creates characteristic facies with frontal bossing, maxillary hypertrophy and overbite. Due to hemolytic jaundice and consequent hemosiderosis skin is often a green-brown color.

β^+/β^+ - Thalassemia intermedia is a marked decrease in β-Chain production allowing some Hgb A to be produced. The anemia is slightly less severe than Cooley anemia but still significant. Physical findings are very similar.

β/β° - β-thalassemia minor involves production of normal β-globin chains but only from one chromosome. Consequently a mild anemia occurs with splenomegaly and jaundice.

β/β^+ - β-thalassemia trait is generally asymptomatic

Laboratory Findings

Hypochromic microcytic anemia (variable)
Peripheral smear - poikilocytosis, anisocytosis, normoblasts, intracellular inclusions.

Unconjugated hyperbilirubinemia
Increased serum iron
Saturation of TIBC
Increased LDH
Hgb Electrophoresis -   Increased Hgb F (>90% in Cooley anemia)
                          Increased Hgb A_2
                          Absent or decreased Hgb A

Treatment

Patients with $\beta°/\beta°$ thalassemia require repeated transfusions every 4-5 weeks. This chronic iron load in addition to hyperabsorption of dietary iron leads to hemosiderosis. To minimize cardiac, hepatic, pancreatic and gonad complications, chelation therapy with desferoxamine is utilized. Splenectomy is often required. Bone marrow transplantation is the definitive treatment. Less severe forms of thalassemia are not transfusion dependent. $\beta/\beta°$ thalassemia must be carefully distinguished from iron deficiency anemia to avoid inappropriate iron therapy.

Alpha-thalassemias
Pathogenesis

Deletions of α-globin genes on chromosome 16 are the most common causes of α-thalassemias. Four genes are present with four forms of thalassemia identified. Alpha chains are required for Hgb A, Hgb A_2 and Hgb F: therefore production of these normal hemoglobins are affected to varying degrees. Excess β chains form tetramers known as Hgb H, which is very unstable. Excess γ chains (part of Hgb F) form tetramers known as Hgb Barts. Hgb Barts has an extremely high oxygen affinity therefore tissue oxygenation is severely impaired.

Clinical Features

Dependent on specific genetic abnormality. Genetic defects found in areas endemic for *Plasmodium falaciparum* malaria (eg, Africa and Southeast Asia).

α-thalassemia major - deletion of all 4 α genes. Hgb Barts is predominate. Incompatible with life with most affected patients dying in utero with hydrops fetalis.

α-thalassemia intermedia - deletion of 3 α genes. Hgb H comprises 4-20% of childhood hemoglobin. Lifelong moderate to severe anemia with hemolysis, splenomegaly and cholecystitis.

α-thalassemia minor - deletion of 2 α genes. Demonstrates as a mild anemia which is commonly confused with iron deficiency anemia.

α-thalassemia carrier - deletion of 1 α gene with no abnormal clinical manifestations.

Laboratory Findings

Hypochromic microcytic anemia (variable)

Unconjugated hyperbilirubinemia

Peripheral smear - intracellular inclusions (unstable hemoglobin)

Elevated Hgb Barts and/or Hgb H

Treatment

Supportive care with transfusions, splenectomy and infection precautions.

Polycythemia

Polycythemia refers to an absolute increase in red blood cell volume, red blood cell count, hemoglobin and hematocrit. Care must be taken to determine if elevations of hematocrit are from the polycythemia or hemoconcentration. Expansion of plasma volume with rehydration corrects hemoconcentration.

Erythrocytosis

Overproduction of RBCs is most commonly secondary to an increased production of erythropoietin. This occurs in any situation associated with hypoxia such as cyanotic congenital heart disease, pulmonary disease, congenital methemoglobinemia, infants of diabetic mothers, small gestational age infants or living at high altitudes. The resultant hyperviscosity may cause thrombosis.

Clinical Features

Newborns often exhibit a ruddy complexion and neurologic abnormalities. Older children exhibit clubbing, cyanosis and hyperemia of mucous membranes.

Laboratory Findings

Newborns - Central hematocrit > 65%

Children - Hematocrit > 55%

Treatment

In the newborn period a partial exchange transfusion is indicated. Whole blood is removed and replaced with saline or albumin to achieve a hematocrit of 50%. The following formula is used for calculations:

$$\text{Vol. of Exchange} = \text{Blood Vol. of Pt.} \times \frac{\text{Observed - Desired Hct}}{\text{Observed Hct}}$$

In older children periodic phlebotomies with saline replacement are also utilized.

Polycythemia Rubra Vera

This is a very rare disorder of childhood. Primary defect is in bone marrow hematopoietic stem cells with marked overproduction of all cell lines. In vitro, RBC precursors are active even without erythropoietin stimulation.

Coagulation Disorders

Blood must maintain an equilibrium between the forces that control hemorrhage and protect against thromboses. This dynamic balance consists of blood vessels, platelets, protein clotting factors and inhibitors. Abnormalities in blood vessels and/or platelets typically results in petechiae, small ecchymoses or mucous membrane bleeding such as epistaxis, hematuria or menorrhagia. Abnormalities in protein factors classically results in deep hemorrhage into muscles and joints.

Abnormalities of Protein Factors

Factor VIII Deficiency (Hemophilia A)

Pathogenesis

A cascade of reactions involving plasma proteins assists in coagulation by forming a stable fibrin clot. If a protein is missing or defective the cascade is ineffective and bleeding occurs with even trivial trauma. An X-linked deficeincy of Factor VIII accounts for 80% of all hemophilias. Severity of bleeding depends on the degree of factor activity. Severe bleeding occurs with < 1% normal activity. Mild disease occurs with 6-30% of normal factor activity.

Clinical Features

Newborn males may present with hematomas after injections or excessive bleeding with circumcision. Most patients will present in the first year of life as ambulation begins and minor trauma occurs. The hallmark of hemophilia is hemorrhage into large joints such as knees and elbows. Repeated hemarthroses may lead to a fixed nonmobile joint. Intracranial hemorrhages are life-threatening emergencies. Family history is helpful.

Laboratory Findings

Prolonged PTT

Mixing study - PTT corrects

Decreased Factor VIII activitty

Normal platelets, PT and bleeding time.

Treatment

Prevention of trauma is the cornerstone of care. Medications that affect platelet function (eg, NSAIDS) should be avoided. Episodes of hemorrhage are managed by replacement with Factor VIII concentrates.

Factor IX Deficiency (Hemophilia B)

Pathogenesis

X-linked recessive deficiency of Factor IX interrupting the clotting cascade. Severity determined by % activity of normal.

Clinical Features

Rarely diagnosed in newborn period as Factor IX levels are low even in normal infants at birth. Otherwise manifestations are virtually identical to Factor VIII deficiency.

Laboratory Findings

Prolonged PTT

Mixing study - PTT corrects

Decreased Factor IX activity

Normal platelets, PT and bleeding time.

Treatment

Avoidance of trauma and anti-platelet medication is important for prevention. Episodes of hemorrhage are managed by replacement with Factor IX concentrates.

von Willebrand Disease

Pathogenesis

Autosomal dominant abnormality of production of function of von Willebrand protein. This protein contains a platelet-adhesive component and serves to carry Factor VIII. Abnormalities lead to abnormal platelet adhesion function and effective decrease in Factor VIII activity.

Clinical Features

Episodes of bleeding are usually related to abnormality of platelet function manifesting as menorrhagia, epistaxis or gingival hemorrhage.

Laboratory Findings
> Prolonged PTT
> Prolonged bleeding time
> Decreased Factor VIII activity
> Normal platelets, PT

Treatment
> Replacement of von Willebrand factor with cryoprecipitate for episodes of hemorrhage. Replacement with Factor VIII concentrate alone does not remedy the effects of abnormal platelet adhesiveness.

Vitamin K Deficiency
> See Hemorrhagic Disease of the Newborn in Chapter 2

Disseminated Intravascular Coagulation

Pathogenesis
> Widespread intravascular activation of the clotting cascade and fibrinolytic system. Initiated by systemic insults such as septic shock, neoplasms, snake envenomation or trauma. Coagulation factors, specifically II, V, VIII and fibrinogen are consumed. In addition hemolytic anemia and thrombocytopenia are present.

Clinical Features
> Symptoms of inciting disease are most notable; however, bleeding from incisions or venipuncture sites is common. Intravascular deposition of fibrin leads to tissue infarction manifesting from purpura fulminans to multi-organ system failure.

Laboratory Findings
> Prolonged PT, PTT, bleeding time
> Decreased fibrinogen
> Elevated fibrin degradation products (FDP)
> Thrombocytopenia
> Normochromic normocytic anemia
> Peripheral smear - fragmented burr cells

Treatment
> Management of inciting insult is imperative. Hemorrhagic abnormalities are managed by replacement therapy with cryoprecipitate, fresh-frozen plasma, platelets and red blood cells as needed.

Abnormalities of Platelets
Inherited Thrombocytopenias
Wiskott-Aldrich Syndrome
Pathogenesis
X-linked recessive defect in platelet formation despite normal megakaryocytes.
Clinical Features
Syndrome association with eczema and recurrent infections. Splenomegaly, hepatomegaly and cervical lymphadenopathy is common.
Laboratory Findings
Thrombocytopenia
Peripheral smear - small platelets
Bone marrow - normal megakaryocytes
Treatment
Splenectomy improves thrombocytopenia but increases the risk of infection. Bone marrow transplantation has been successful.

Thrombocytopenia Absent Radius (TAR) Syndrome
Pathogenesis
Autosomal recessive absence of bone marrow megakaryocytes.
Clinical Features
Syndromic association with absent radii. Cardiac and renal abnormalities are often associated findings.
Laboratory Findings
Profound thrombocytopenia
Normal chromosome configuration
Bone marrow - absent megakaryocytes
Treatment
Supportive platelet transfusions as needed.

Kasabach-Merritt Syndrome
Pathogenesis
Cavernous hemangromas of the trunk, extremities and viscera are sites of intravascular coagulation and subsequent thrombocytopenia.
Clinical Features
Hemangiomas may or may not be visible. Recurrent symptoms of thrombocytopenia and anemia occur.

Laboratory Findings

Thrombocytopenia

Peripheral smear - red blood cell fragments

Bone marrow - normal megakaryocytes

Treatment

Reduction of hemangioma size can be attempted with surgical excision, radiation therapy, coritcosteroids &/or interferon. Platelet and PRBC transfusions are given as needed for supportive care.

Acquired Thrombocytopenia

Idiopathic Thrombocytopenic Purpura (ITP)

Pathogenesis

Ill-defined etiology; however often associated with a preceding viral illness. Likely an immune mechanism triggers platelet destruction.

Clinical Features

Acute onset of petechiae, epistaxis, gingival hemorrhage is noted about 2 weeks after a viral illness. Patient appears clinically normal except for hemorrhage. Intracranial hemorrhages are very rare.

Laboratory Findings

Thrombocytopenia

Bone marrow - increased megakaryocytes suggestive of increased platelet production.

Treatment

Episodes of life-threatening hemorrhage require platelet transfusions; however transfused platelets are rapidly destroyed as well. Spontaneous recovery within 8 weeks is expected but this can be hastened with intravenous gamma globulin or steroid therapy. Some patients experience prolonged thrombocytopenia called chronic ITP if > 1 year. These patients may benefit from splenectomy.

Veena Khanna

Developmental Considerations

The gastrointestinal tract is formed during the fourth week of gestation in the form of a small 4 mm hollow tube. The epithelial tissues of the gut are derived from the endodermal layer, whereas the muscles and connective tissues are derived from the mesodermal layer of the embryo during invagination of the embryonic disc. Foregut comprises the esophagus, stomach, duodenum, liver, gallbladder and pancreas. The midgut is composed of jejunum, ileum and the ascending and transverse colon, and the hindgut comprises the descending and rectosigmoid colon.

During the first two trimesters of pregnancy, several major events occur. The third trimester is the period of maximal intrauterine growth and differentiation of the gastrointestinal tract.

The three major physiological functions are:
- Motility
- Absorption and secretion
- Immunologic protection.

Some gut functions develop early in fetal life, but others mature postnatally and some are not fully developed until preschool age. The uniqueness of the human gut is seen in its ability to adapt to a variety of nutrient sources and to utilize them for further growth and development.

Common GI problems seen in the newborn include:

Cleft Lip/Palate
Cleft lip appears to be due to hypoplasia of the mesenchymal layer resulting in failure of medial nasal and maxillary processes to join. Cleft of the palate appears to represent failure of the palatal shelves to approximate or fuse.

Incidence of cleft lip with or without cleft palate is about 1:1000, and of cleft palate alone is 1:2500. Genetic factors are more important in cleft lip; the incidence is highest among Asians and lowest among Blacks. The recurrence risk is 3-4% in siblings.

Treatment initially is focused on feeding with the aid of plastic obturator and soft artificial nipples with large holes. Surgical closure of cleft lip is performed by 2 months after adequate weight gain. It can be revised at 4-5 years of age. Timing of correction of cleft palate is individualized, and usually done prior to 1 year of age.

Complications are ear infections, hearing loss, dental decay, malocclusions, and speech defects.

Management requires multidisciplinary approach.

Pierre Robin Syndrome

This sequence consists of micrognathia with glossoptosis and pseudomacroglossia with high arched or cleft palate (partial).

Obstruction of the air passages may occur particularly on inspiration and usually requires therapy to prevent suffocation. Feeding problems may occur. Often the mandibular growth will achieve an essentially natural profile within 4-6 years.

Esophageal Atresia

This generally occurs in association with tracheo-esophagal fistula. The most common anatomic arrangement is a blind proximal esophageal pouch that has a distal TE-fistula (85-90%). Incidence of this anomaly is 1 in 4000. Associated anomalies occur in 40% of EA.

The presentation is usually excessive drooling, regurgitation, cough, choking, or cyanosis with feeding. Abdominal distention or scaphoid abdomen may occur depending on fistulous connection.

Diagnosis is by radiography. Primary repair can be done in babies as small as 1200 g. Child with complications such as aspiration pneumonia or with pure EA need staged repair. Progress is usually excellent but complications like stricture formation at anastomotic site can easily be managed with dilatation.

Omphalocele

This is usually associated with a high incidence of other malformations (namely congenital heart disease or Beckwith-Wiedemann Syndrome).

Omphalocele is herniation of abdominal contents into the base of the umbilical cord, the sac being covered by peritoneum only. Treatment is surgical.

Umbilical Hernia

More common in premature and black infants

Increased incidence in hypothyroidism

Fascial defects less than 0.5 cm usually spontaneously close by age 2 years; defects 0.5-1.5 cm spontaneously close by age 4 years.

Abdominal binders (coins, etc. taped over defect) do not increase healing rate.

Duodenal Obstruction
May be due to atresia (complete obstruction) or stenosis (partial obstruction due to a web, band, or annular pancreas) in the neonate.

More common in premature and infants with Down syndrome.

Jejunal/Ileal Obstruction
Meconium ileus with or without atresia is associated with cystic fibrosis.

Polyhydramnios is present in complete atresia.

Bile-stained vomitus within 24-48 hours after feeding.

X-ray of the abdomen shows dilated loops of small bowel, with absence of air in the colon.

Malrotation/Volvulus
The majority of infants with this anomaly present with symptoms within the first month of life.

Bilious vomiting and abdominal distention suggests obstruction.

Bloody stools may occur if volvulus results in bowel ischemia.

Meckel's Diverticulum
The most common anomaly of the gastrointestinal tract.

It is due to the presence of a vestigial remnant of the omphalomesenteric duct.

Gastric tissue is common in symptomatic cases because it causes acid secretion and ulceration.

Presenting clinical manifestations include: painless rectal bleeding, intestinal obstruction (due to intussusception or volvulus) or diverticulitis (mimics appendicitis).

Rule of '2's"
- in 2 % population
- a 2:1 male-to-female ratio
- is 2" long
- has 2 tissues; gastric and pancreatic
- is 2 ft proximal to ileocecal valve
- has 2 bimodal presentations; < 2 years old and adolescence
- have 2 presentations; hemorrhage, obstruction

Diagnostic Modalities

History
- Pain
- Vomiting
- Weight loss
- Stools (frequency, color, blood, consistency, smell)

Physical Examination
- General appearance
- Growth
- Oral mucosa
- Teeth (eruption pattern, enamel, caries)
- Abdominal tenderness
- Organomegaly
- Bowel sounds
- Rectal (anus patent, stool, blood)

"Red Flags" on Physical Examination

- Documented weight loss
- Abdominal wall hernia
- Organomegaly
- Perianal fistula
- Anal fissure
- Perirectal ulceration
- Occult blood in the stool
- Joint swelling and tenderness
- Ophthalmologic signs of systemic involvement of gastrointestinal disease

Laboratory

Which lab is appropriate must be guided strongly by history and exam results:
- CBC
- Sedimentation rate
- Amylase
- Serum chemistries
- Hemoccult
- Stool for ova and parasites
- Hydrogen breath testing

Sweat chloride
Urinalysis
Stool culture (bacterial, viral)
Stool pH and reducing substance
Stool for fecal fat
Esophageal pH study

Radiographic and Other Studies

Again, what is appropriate depends on the patient's age, history and exam:

Abdominal X-ray
Abdominal ultrasound
Endoscopy
Barium enema
Meckel's scan
Barium swallow
Chest X-ray

Pathophysiologic Manifestations

Common Causes of Abdominal Pain by Age

Infant	Child	Adolescent
Necrotizing enterocolitis	Gastroenteritis	Pelvic inflammatory disease
Volvulus	Appendicitis	Ectopic pregnancy
Incarcerated hernia	Henoch-Schönlein purpura	Inflammatory bowel disease
Hirschsprung's disease	Urinary tract infection	Testicular torsion
Intussusception	Hemolytic-Uremic syndrome	Biliary disease
Infantile colic	Constipation	
Perforation (R/O abuse)	Ulcers	
	Pancreatitis	
	Functional pain/recurrent abdominal pain	

"Red Flags" in the History of Abdominal Pain

- Pain well localized away from the umbilicus (Apley's Law*)
- Changes in bowel function (constipation, diarrhea, incontinence)
- Vomiting
- Sudden onset of constant pain that lasts minutes to days
- Pain that awakens child at night
- Pain that radiates to back, shoulder, or lower extremities
- Dysuria
- Rectal bleeding
- Constitutional symptoms (fever, weight loss, altered rate of growth, rash, arthralgia)
- Presentation at < 4 years or > 15 years of age
- Family history of gastrointestinal or systemic illness (peptic ulcer disease, inflammatory bowel disease)

The further the pain from the umbilicus, the more likely that it represents identifiable disease.

Pathophysiologic Mechanisms of Diarrhea

Mechanism	Pathophysiology	Stool Characteristics
Secretory	decreased absorption; increased secretion	Watery; Normal osmolality: osmols = 2 X $(Na^+ + K^+)$
Osmotic	Maldigestion; transport Watery; defects	Acidic: + reducing substances; Increased osmolality: osmols > 2 X $(Na^+ + K^+)$
Increased peristalsis	Decreased transient time	Fecal-like; Stimulated by gastrocolic reflex
Decreased mucosal area	Decreased functional capacity	Watery
Mucosal invasion	Inflammation; decreased colonic reabsorption; increased motility	Blood and increased WBC

Differential Diagnosis of Constipation

	NEWBORN	INFANT	TODDLER AND SCHOOL-AGE CHILD
MECHANICAL OBSTRUCTION	Imperforate or stenotic anus (sometimes with VATER syndrome) Intestinal atresia Small left colon syndrome Meconium ileus Meconium plug Tumor	Anterior ectopic anus Tumors (lymphoma, rhabdomyosarcoma, neuroblastoma) Malrotation Rectal duplications Congenital or acquired strictures or adhesive peritoneal bands	Tumors (lymphoma, rhabdomyosarcoma, neuroblastoma) Malrotation Rectal duplications Congenital or acquired strictures or adhesive peritoneal bands Crohn disease
OTHER INTESTINAL DISEASE	Hirschsprung disease Neuronal intestinal dysplasias Primary ganglioneuromatosis Visceral myopathies and neuropathies	Hirschsprung disease Visceral myopathies and neuropathies von Recklinghausen disease Multiple endocrine neoplasia type IIB Myotonic dystrophy	Hirschsprung disease Multiple endocrine neoplasia type IIB Myotonic dystrophy Dermatomyositis
ABNORMALITY OUTSIDE THE GASTROINTESTINAL TRACT	Hypothyroidism Adrenal insufficiency Hyper- or hypokalemia Hypercalcemia Hypermagnesemia	Spinal cord lesion Familial dysautonomia Hypothyroidism Hypokalemia Hypercalcemia Infant botulism Drug-induced constipation	Spinal cord lesion Autonomic neuropathy, primary or acquired Lead poisoning Drug-induced constipation Hypothyroidism Hypokalemia Hypercalcemia Porphyria Pheochromocytoma Diabetes mellitus
FUNCTIONAL DISORDER	None	Dietary abnormality Slow transit	Dietary abnormality Functional fecal retention

Comparison of Functional Fecal Retention and Hirschsprung Disease

SYMPTOM	FUNCTIONAL FECAL RETENTION	HIRSCHSPRUNG DISEASE
Delayed meconium passage	Rare	60%
Constipation as newborn	Rare	Almost always
Onset after age 2 years	Common	Sometimes
Fecal incontinence	Common	Almost never
Difficult bowel training	Common	Rare
Avoidance of toilet	Common	Rare
Withholding behavior	Common	Rare
Stool in rectal ampulla	Common	Rare
Obstructive symptoms	Rare	Common

Disease Profiles

Gastroesophageal Reflux
This is a common problem seen in the first year of life. Passive reflux of gastric contents causes symptoms if the lower esophageal sphincter is incompetent. The incidence of significant reflux and complications is 1:300 to 1:10,000.

Mechanics
- Lax LES (lower esophogeal sphincter) or brief but frequent spontaneous decreases in sphincter tone
- Increased intraabdominal pressure
- Decreased gastric emptying
- Reduced esophageal acid clearance

Symptoms
- Vomiting in infants - abates by age 2 years in 60% of cases without treatment.
- GI bleeding
- Aspiration pneumonia
- Apnea (Apparent Life-Threatening Event)
- Failure to thrive

Diagnosis
- History
- UGI series under fluoroscopy
- 24 hours esophageal pH monitoring
- Gastric scintigrams

Management
- Uncomplicated Case
  * head end elevated (30 degrees)
  * thickening formula with cereal
  * frequent burping
- Complicated
  * antacids/H$_2$ - blockers for esophagitis
  * motility agents - Metoclopramide or Cisapride.
  * surgery (Nissen Fundoplication if medical treatment fails)

Pyloric Stenosis

Occurs usually in males (1:150) and is associated with nonbilious projectile vomiting beginning at 2-4 weeks of age. Multifactorial inheritance is likely but it sometimes occurs in mini-epidemics.

Etiology

Unknown

Association

Diffuse hypertrophy and hyperplasia of pyloric sphincter muscle as well as involvement of antral muscle. Prolonged vomiting gives rise to failure to thrive, gastritis with or without hemorrhage, electrolyte imbalance (metabolic, hypokalemic alkalosis) and occasionally hyperbilirubinemia.

Characteristic Symptoms

Gradual onset of nonbilous vomiting progressing to projectile episodes. The baby is hungry and will feed voraciously even right after the vomiting episodes.

Diagnosis
>Careful history
>Palpation of "olive" (successful palpation requires a vast amount of patience, a relaxed anterior abdominal wall and an empty stomach)
>Confirmation may be done by ultrasound examination of pylorus or barium studies.

Management
>Correction of electrolyte and acid-base abnormalities followed by surgical relief. Nonsurgical treatment with cholinergic blocking agent has been virtually abandoned.

Hirschprung Disease
Due to the absence of intramural neural ganglia in the rectum leading to constipation.

Pathogenesis
>Current research suggests that Hirschprung disease results from arrest of migration of vagal neural crest cells due to abnormalities of the extracellular matrix of distal bowel. Extrinsic nerve axonal processes still enter the bowel, proliferate and stimulate unopposed contraction resulting in functional obstruction of the aganglionic bowel segment.

Epidemiology
>Rare, with an incidence of 1:5000 live births. Males are predominantly affected (80%). A family history can be obtained in 7% of cases. Risk of disease to sibling of affected patient is 2.5%.

Association
>Waardenburg's syndrome
>Smith-Lemli-Opitz Syndrome
>Trisomy 21
>13 Short arm Deletion Syndrome

Presentation
>In newborn:
>>Delayed passage of meconium
>>Constipation in first several days
>>Intestinal obstruction
>In infant:
>>Constipation
>>Enterocolitis (toxic megacolon)

Diagnosis
>Unprepped barium enema examination - reveals a small distal colon with a dilated segment above the 'transition zone'.

Anorectal manometry - evaluates response of anal sphincter to inflation of a balloon in the rectum (negative response in Hirschsprung disease).

Rectal biopsy

Management

The only safe and effective treatment is surgical.

Diarrhea

Gastroenteritis both acute and chronic may occur as often as 15 times per year in a child. In the U.S. attack rates average 1.3 to 2.3 episodes per year between ages 0 and 5 years; incidence peaking in winters.

Causes

Acute Diarrhea

Local infection - noninvasive

Rotavirus

Norwalk virus

Enteric adenovirus

Giardia lamblia

Crytosporidium

Esherichia coli

Systemic infections - invasive or toxigenic

Campylobacter jejunii

Salmonella

Shigella

Yersinnia

Escherichia coli

Clostridium difficile

Chronic Diarrhea

Self-limited - nonspecific diarrhea

Pathologic diarrhea

Congenital

Enzyme deficiencies

Enterokinase

Sucrase-isomaltose

Glucose-galactose

Chloridorrhea

Microvillus atrophy

Short gut

Acquired
    Postinfectious
    Infectious
        Parasitic
        $2°$ to immunodeficiency
        Bacterial overgrowth
    Malabsorption, maldigestion
    Intestinal
        Inflammatory bowel disease
        Protein-losing enteropathy; milk allergy
        Disaccharidase deficiency
        Short gut
        Autoimmune microvillus atrophy
    Exocrine pancreas
        Cystic fibrosis
        Schwachmann syndrome
        Chronic pancreatitis
    Liver
        Bile acid deficiencies, either $1°$ or $2°$ to
            cholestatic syndromes
    Drugs
        Laxatives
        Sorbitol
        Antacids
        Antibiotics
    Miscellaneous
        Endocrine tumors
        Heavy metal poisoning

Acute Diarrhea
    Investigations
        Stool consistency, fecal leukocytes
        Stools for bacterial cultures, virology, ova and parasites
        Blood chemistry if indicated
    Management
        Hydration
            Oral fluids
            Intravenous fluids

Early refeeding advisable
Antidiarrheal drugs rarely indicated
Specific treatment
      C difficile → Vancomycin, Metronidazole
      Shigella → Amoxicillin, Cotrimoxazole
      Campylobacter → Erythromycin
      Giardia → Metronidazole, Furazolidone
      Yersinnia → Cotrimoxazole, Chloramphenicol, Tetracycline (> age
         9 yr)

Persistent Diarrhea

By definition persistent (or chronic) diarrhea lasts longer than 14 days.

Investigations

Serial heights and weights
Stool examination - consistency, pH, reducing substances, fecal leukocytes,
    blood, fat globules, ova and parasites, cultures
Stool collection
    fat malabsorption → 3-day fecal fat
    protein malabsorption → alpha-1 antitrypsin clearance,
        electrolytes
Blood - CBC with diff., ESR, electrolytes, BUN, creatinine, protein,
    immunoglobulins, chemistry (CA, PO_4, Fe, folate, vitamins, liver
    function, PT, PTT, etc), HIV, lead
Urine - urinalysis, cultures, HVA, VMA
Breath hydrogen
Sweat test
Radiological examinations - upper GI series ± follow through, barium
    enema (double contrast)
Specialized tests
    small bowel biopsy
    endoscopy
    quantitative exocrine pancreatic testing

Management

Nonspecific diarrhea of infancy (toddler's diarrhea) requires no specific
therapy. Fruit juices should be avoided. In postinfectious diarrhea,
although no specific therapy is indicated, adequate protein and caloric
replacement factors most in its resolution.

Specific therapy is required for other etiologies:

Disease	Treatment
Enterokinase deficiency	Protein hydrolysate formula (infants), pancreatic enzyme replacement
Short gut, microvillus atrophy	± Parenteral nutrition, consider somatostatin analogues, prednisone (autoimmune etiology)
Protein-losing enteropathy	Depends on underlying disorder
Bacterial overgrowth	Poorly absorbed antibiotics, eg, metronidazole, gentamicin
Inflammatory bowel disease	Drugs, elemental diet
Exocrine pancreatic insufficiency	Titrated pancreatic enzyme replacement, fat-soluble vitamin, ↑ calories (120-150% of recommended daily intake)
Lactase deficiency	Lactase additives, avoid lactose-containing products
Celiac disease	Gluten-free diet

Encopresis
See Chapter 4

Recurrent Abdominal Pain
See Chapter 4

Chronic Inflammatory Bowel Disease
Chronic inflammatory bowel disease can be either Crohn's disease or Ulcerative colitis. The cause is unknown but probably due to an immunologically-mediated chronic inflammatory response in a genetically susceptible host. It begins in late childhood or adolescence with bloody diarrhea, abdominal cramps, weight loss or growth failure. Extra-intestinal manifestations occur more frequently in Crohn's disease (regional ileitis).

Comparison

Feature	Crohn Ds	U. Colitis
Rectal bleeding	±	+
Rectal disease	±	++
Abdominal mass	+	-
Ileal disease	+	-
Perianal disease	+	-
Strictures/fistula	+	-
Skip lesions	+	-
Transmural disease	+	-
Crypt abscesses	-	+
Granulomas	+	-
Colon cancer risk	±	++

Differential Diagnosis
Infections
Bacterial: *Yersinia, Campylobacter, Salmonella, Shigella,* Tuberculosis
Parasitic: *E. histolytica, Giardia*
HIV related: Cryptosporidium, CMV
Immunologic
Immunodeficiency: congenital, acquired
Behçet's syndrome
Lymphoid nodular hyperplasia
Graft-versus-Host disease
Vasculitis
Systemic Lupus Erythematosus
Henoch-Schönlein Purpura
Hemolytic-Uremic Syndrome
Malignancy
Lymphoma
Adenocarcinoma
Investigations
See malabsorption
Treatment
Nutritional support
Supportive care
Pharmacotherapy
Surgery

Gastrointestinal Bleeding

Causes of Upper Gastrointestinal Bleeding by Age Group

Neonate	Infant	Child	Adolescent
Swallowed maternal blood	Gastritis	Esophageal varices	Esophageal varices
Gastritis	Esophagitis	Peptic ulcer disease	Peptic ulcer
Esophagitis	Stress ulcer	Stress ulcer	Gastritis
Congenital blood dyscrasia	Mallory-Weiss tear	Gastritis	Mallory-Weiss tear
Vascular malformation	Duplication	Mallory-Weiss tear	Esophagitis
	Vascular malformation	Foreign body	Stress ulcer
		Esophagitis	

Causes of Lower Gastrointestinal Bleeding by Age Group

Neonate	Infant	Child	Adolescent
Anal fissure	Anal fissure	Polyps	Polyps
Upper GI bleeding	Intussusception	Anal fissure	Hemorrhoids
Volvulus	Meckel's diverticulum	Meckel's diverticulum	Inflammatory bowel disease
Necrotizing enterocolitis	Infectious diarrhea	Infectious diarrhea	Infectious diarrhea
Swallowed maternal blood	Milk allergy	Henoch-Schönlein Purpura	
Infectious colitis	Duplication	Hemolytic-Uremic Syndrome	
Milk allergy	Pseudomembranous colitis	Intussusception	
Blood dyscrasia		Pseudomembranous colitis	
Duplication			

Infectious Causes of Hematochezia
Salmonella
Shigella
Yersina
Campylobacter
Enterohemorrhagic *E coli*
Enteroinvasive *E coli*
Clostridium difficile
Entamoeba histolytica

Investigations
Blood - CBC, hematocrit, differential, ESR PT, PTT, BUN, Creatinine, liver functions.
Stool - gross and microscopy for leukocytes, occult blood, cultures.
Radiological investigations - upper GI ± follow through. Barium enema (single contrast for obstruction; double contrast for mucosal abnormalities) or plain abdominal X-rays to rule out obstruction.
Specialized tests
Diagnostic endoscopy ± biopsy
Meckel's scan
Angiography
^{99} TeRBC scan (bleeding scan)

Management
Initial stabilization - volume and blood replacement, NG suction, NPO.

Therapeutic Modalities
Lavage with therapeutic endoscopy
Intravascular injection of vasoactive agents eg, Vasopressin, Somatostatin
Balloon Tamponade
Sclerotherapy
Thermal coagulation
Electrocoagulation
Laser photocoagulation

Malabsorptive Disorders
These are disorders that lead to defective assimilation of nutrients, and manifesting with abdominal distension; pale, foul, bulky stools; retardation of height and weight, and muscle weakness.
Causes
Defective Digestion

Pancreatic Deficiency
 cystic fibrosis
 pancreatitis
 Schwachmann syndrome
Bile Salt Deficiency
 biliary atresia
 cholestasis
 hepatitis
 cirrhosis
 bacterial deconjugation
Defective Absorption
 Primary Absorption Defects
 glucose-galactose malabsorption
 abetalipoproteinemia
 cystinuria
 Hartnup disease
 Decreased Mucosal Surface Area
 Crohn disease
 malnutrition
 short bowel syndrome
 Small Intestinal Disease
 Celiac disease
 tropical sprue
 giardiasis
 lymphoma
 allergic enteritis
 Infestations
 hookworm
 tapeworm
 opportunistic infections in AIDS
 Lymphatic Obstruction
 lymphangiectasia
 Whipple disease
 lymphoma
Laboratory Evaluation
 Microbiology - *Giardia*
 Hematology - CBC, differential, blood, film (hypochromia, microcytosis,
  macrocytosis, acanthocytes, leukopenia)
 Chemistry - liver function, vitamins, serum carotene, protein,
  immunoglobulins

Absorptive function
      Fat $\rightarrow$ fecal fat
                             fasting serum carotene
                             stool for fat globules
      Carbohydrate $\rightarrow$ stool for reducing substances
                             breath for hydrogen test
      Protein $\rightarrow$ Enteric protein loss measurement
                             Fecal alpha-1 antitrypsin clearance
      Nutrients in blood $\rightarrow$ Fe, Ca, Vit., A, D, B_{12}
      Xylose absorption test - to localize site of lesion
      Schilling test - for B_{12} absorption
      Quantitative pancreatic function testing
Imaging
      Plain X-rays
      Barium studies
      Ultrasound
      Retrograde pancreatic and biliary tree studies
Biopsy and endoscopy

A Eugene Osburn

Developmental Considerations

Nephrogenesis is not complete until 36 weeks gestation. Therefore, premature infants have compromised renal functional capacity compared to term infants.

Fetal urine is excreted into the amniotic fluid. Oligohydramnios will result from inadequate urine output from a fetus.

Inadequate amniotic fluid is associated with pulmonary hypoplasia which may be incompatible with life.

Potter's syndrome, which is characterized by a typical facial appearance, low set ears and pulmonary hypoplasia can be a result of severe intrauterine oliguria or anuria.

Intrauterine urinary tract obstruction can cause renal dysplasia with resulting renal insufficiency from which the infant may not completely recover.

Serum Creatinine for the first 5 days of life in the newborn reflects the mother's creatinine level, not the infant's renal function.

Glomerular filtration rate: The GFR at birth is 20 to 30 ml/1.73 m^2/min.
     The GFR doubles (40 to 60) by 2 weeks after birth.
     The GFR should reach adult levels (120 ml/1.73m^2/min.) by age 2 years.

Clearance of drugs cleared by renal excretion may cause toxicity if given to infants in doses based on expected adult level GFR.

Urine concentrating and diluting ability: Newborn kidneys can only concentrate urine to 1/2 that of adults. ie, 600-700 mosm/kg, instead of 1200-1400 mosm/kg. Newborns can dilute urine to adult levels (50 mosm/kg), but total water load excretion is limited by decreased GFRs.

Electrolyte regulation: Newborns can neither conserve nor effectively excrete excess sodium. As a result, potassium and hydrogen secretion are impaired.

Diagnostic Modalities

Urinalysis

Specific Gravity

1.002 reflects a maximally dilute urine and correlates with a urine osmolality of 50 mosm/kg. 1.035 (1200 mosm/kg osmolality) reflects maximally concentrated urine. Isosthenuria, or a specific gravity of 10.10 (osmolality of 300 mosm/kg), reflects neither concentration nor dilution of filtered serum.

Urine Dipsticks

Commonly available dipsticks measure albumin, glucose, ketones, bilirubin, blood, and leukocyte esterase. Positive blood in the absence of RBCs in the microscopic occurs from free hemoglobin and myoglobin in the urine.

Urine Microscopy

Useful for identifying RBCs WBCs, casts, crystals and bacteria. The presence of epithelial cells should also be noted since large numbers may reflect a non-clean catch specimen. The urine must be examined as soon as possible after voiding to accurately identify microscopic components since cells and casts can lyse in urine.

Urine Electrolytes

Sodium

Maximal conservation is reflected by a value of < 20 mEq/L.
In renal failure the urine sodium is > 50 mEq/L.

Chloride

Maximum conservation is reflected by a value < 10 mEq/L.
The significance of urine chloride concentrations must be interpreted in light of the patient's acid-base status.

Potassium

Maximal tubular conservation is reflected in a value of < 20 mEq/L. Low values may reflect a total body deficit of potassium, regardless of the serum potassium level, although the urine potassium also reflects renin activity and tubular response to that activity. Increased renin activity, (whether physiologically or pathologically elevated) will increase potassium excretion. Renin can be elevated in response to hypovolemic states even in presence of total body or serum potassium deficits.

Glomerular Function Tests

Blood Urea Nitrogen (BUN)

Dependent on dietary protein intake.

Begins to rise when GFR < 50% normal.

Elevation also caused by blood in GI tract.

Upon restoration of normal renal function, elevated BUN levels should decrease by 1/2 it's level every 16 hours.

Serum Creatinine (Cr)

Not influenced by protein intake. The normal value can be estimated by the formula: Cr = 0.004 x height in centimeters.

BUN/Cr Ratio

Normal: 15:1 (range 10:1 to 20:1)

Prerenal azotemia: > 40:1

Glomerular Filtration Rate (GFR)

The most common method used for measuring the GFR is by calculating the Creatinine Clearance (C_{Cr}).

Creatinine Clearance (C_{Cr}) calculation:

$$C_{Cr} = \frac{\text{Urine Cr x Urine Volume}}{\text{Plasma Cr}}$$

$$\text{Corrected } C_{Cr} = \frac{\text{Patient's } C_{Cr} \text{ x } 1.73 \text{ m}^2}{\text{Patient's surface area}}$$

$$\text{Simplified } C_{Cr} = \frac{\text{K x Height in cm}}{\text{Plasma Cr in mg/dl}}$$

K = 0.45 under 1 year age

K = 0.55 over 1 year age

Renal Tubular Function Tests

Tubular function tests can help differentiate between causes of oliguria due to decreased GFR in the presence of tubules with normal functional capability (prerenal azotemia) and those accompanied by more diffuse renal damage (renal failure azotemia). In prerenal azotemia the FEN_a is low (< 1%), whereas, in renal failure azotemia, it is high (> 7%).

Fractional excretion of sodium (FENa) calculation:

$$FENa = \frac{\text{urine Na} \times \text{serum Cr}}{\text{urine Cr} \times \text{serum Na}} \times 100\%$$

Imaging Tests
Ultrasound
Non-invasive. It can identify the size, shape, and density of the kidneys, but is not helpful for assessing renal function.

Intravenous Pyelography
Should rarely be used in children since the availability of radionuclide scanning. Besides the potential of allergic reactions to the dye, it's tonicity can precipitate renal failure. It does provide better delineation of caliceal structures than radionuclide scans.

Voiding Cystourethrography
Useful for identifying vesicoureteral reflux. The same information can be obtained more safely with radionuclide scanning, except for visualization of the urethra.

Radionuclide Scanning
Can provide as assessment of GFR in each kidney as well as assessment of tubular activity depending on which isotope is used. When instilled into the bladder instead of being given IV, it can be used for cystograms, but not visualization of the urethra.

Serum Complement (C₃)
Hypocomplementemia can be found in the following conditions:

Poststreptococcal glomerulonephritis (should return to normal within 8 weeks)

Systemic lupus erythematosus (decreased complement reflects exacerbation of active lupus nephritis)

Membranoproliferative glomerulonephritis (the complement level remains persistently low)

Chronic infections (decreased complement reflects vasculitis which can involve glomerular artery)

Hereditary complement deficiencies (can also be associated with vasculitis)

Renal Biopsy

May be necessary if a histologic diagnosis is needed. It is generally not needed in uncomplicated cases of Lipoid Nephrosis of Childhood, nor in acute glomerulonephritis.

Indications for Dialysis

In acute renal failure, the level of BUN and/or Creatinine are not the determining factors in deciding when to initiate dialysis.

Dialysis is initiated in acute renal failure to control:
Acidosis
Metabolic
Electrolyte Abnormalities, Especially hyperkalemia (which may not be controlled by diet alone when the GFR drops below 5 ml/min/1.73m^2)
Fluid Overload
Hypertension
Congestive heart failure
Pulmonary edema
Uremic Complications
Encephalopathy
Pericarditis or pericardial effusion
Coagulation disturbances

In chronic renal failure, dialysis will generally be required when the GFR falls to < 0.1-0.15 ml/min/kg (7-11 ml/min/1.73m^2)

Pathophysiologic Manifestations

Oliguria

May be a normal physiologic response to water and/or salt depletion, ie, prerenal oliguria, or a reflection of renal failure. The concomitant presence of azotemia reflects a process beyond the kidney's ability to compensate.

Differentiation of Prerenal vs. Renal Oliguria		
TEST	PRERENAL	RENAL
FEN_a	< 1%	> 3%
BUN/Cr ratio	> 20:1	< 10:1
Urine Specific Gravity	>1.015	<1.010

Edema

Edema formation requires an excessive accumulation of both sodium and salt. The kidneys may cause edema due to ineffective excretion of sodium and water or through their enhanced reabsorption either to replenish a decreased intravascular volume or in response to mineralocorticoid excesses.

Causes of Generalized Edema

Inability to excrete sodium and water load

Glomerular lesions resulting in decreased GFR
Excess salt intake

Loss of plasma oncotic pressure

Nephrotic syndrome
Protein-losing enteropathy
Chronic heart failure

Decreased cardiac output

Congestive heart failure
Pericardial effusion

Excessive mineralocorticoid activity

Hyper-renin states
Hyperaldosteronism
Corticosteroid excess

Hepatic failure

Polyuria

Water conservation is dependent on Antidiuretic Hormone (ADH) and it's effect on end organ sites on the distal renal tubules.

Causes of Polyuria

Central diabetes insipidus (ADH deficiency)

    Idiopathic diabetes insipidus
    Acquired diabetes insipidus

        CNS infections
        Pituitary trauma

Nephrogenic diabetes insipidus (end organ defect)

    Heredity form
    Acquired forms

        Interstitial nephritis
        Sickle cell disease
        Chronic renal failure
        Hypokalemia
        Papillary necrosis

Psychogenic polydipsia
Osmotic loads

    Glucose

        Uncontrolled diabetes mellitus
        Iatrogenic hyperglycemia

    Mannitol

Volume expansion

    IV fluids
    Diuretic phase of resolving acute renal failure

Hypertension

Renal diseases are the most common organic cause of hypertension in children. The finding of hypertension demands evaluation of renal function. Hypertension may be due to salt and water retention, excess renin or both as the result of a renal disease. In general hypertension should be further evaluated if the blood pressure is greater than 120/80 in infants, 140/90 in children or 160/100 in adolescents, or is associated with the following signs of end organ insult:

End Organ	Manifestation of Hypertensive Insult
CNS	Hypertensive encephalopathy, increased intracranial pressure Headache, seizures, altered sensorium
Heart	Congestive heart failure, pulmonary edema, ventricular hypertrophy
Kidney	Proteinuria, decreased GFR

Hematuria

Normal number of RBC/HPF in urine: < 5

Proteinuria

Normal protein excretion: < 4 mg/m^2/hour

Nephrotic syndrome producing rate of protein excretion: > 40 mg/m^2/hour

Differentiating the cause of proteinuria and/or hematuria can be facilitated by consideration of associated findings in the patient:

Proteinuria without hematuria or edema:

Transient proteinuria
Orthostatic proteinuria
"Allergic" phenomena
Pre-nephrotic
Focal segmental glomerulosclerosis

Proteinuria with edema and no hematuria:

Minimal lesion nephrotic syndrome
Focal segmental glomerulosclerosis

Proteinuria with edema and hematuria:

Acute glomerulonephritis
Minimal lesion nephrotic syndrome
Chronic and/or progressive glomerulonephritis

> Lupus Nephritis
> Membranoproliferative glomerulonephritis
> Hereditary glomerulonephritis

Proteinuria with hematuria and no edema:

Acute glomerulonephritis
Idiopathic hypercalciuria
IgA Nephropathy
Reflux nephropathy
Acute interstitial nephritis
Urinary tract infection
Cystic kidneys

Hematuria without proteinuria or edema:

Benign transient hematuria
Trauma
Idiopathic hypercalciuria
Nephrolithiasis
Urethral foreign body

Enuresis

90% of children stop bedwetting by the age of 5 years. Urinary tract infections and idiopathic hypercalcinuria need to be ruled out. Arginine vasopressin (DDAVP) may be useful in some children. Tricylic antidepressants have been used, but have potentially dangerous side effects, and are not recommended.

Nephrotic Syndrome

The nephrotic syndrome is characterized by **proteinuria, hypoproteinemia, edema, and hyperlipidemia.** If urinary protein loss exceeds 40 mg/m²/hour for an adequate length of time, hypoproteinemia (due to the liver's inability to replenish the loss), edema (due to decreased oncotic pressure) and hyperlipidemia (a by-product of the increased liver synthesis of protein) will ensue.

Causes of Nephrotic Syndrome

Primary glomerular involvement

  Without inflammatory glomerular changes

    Minimal change nephrotic syndrome
    Focal segmental glomerulosclerosis
    Congenital nephrotic syndrome

  With inflammatory glomerular changes

    Acute poststreptococcal glomerulonephritis
    Membranoproliferative glomerulonephritis
    Membranous nephropathy
    Mesangial proliferative glomerulonephritis

Glomerular insults secondary to systemic diseases with vasculitis

  Inflammatory diseases

    Systemic lupus erythematosus
    Henoch-Schonlein purpura
    System vasculitis
    Hemolytic-uremia syndrome

Infections

    Viral infections

        Hepatitis
        Cytomegalovirus
        Epstein-Barr virus

    Bacterial infections

        Shunt nephritis
        Subacute bacterial endocarditis

    Parasitic infections

        Malaria

Malignant diseases

    Lymphomas
    Leukemias
    Solid tumors

Metabolic diseases

    Diabetes mellitus
    Hypothyroidism

Exogenous toxins and poisons

    Medications
    Heavy metals
    Venoms

Other disorders

    Sickle cell disease
    Renal vein thrombosis

Renal Failure

May occur with or without decreased urine output, ie, oliguric or non-oliguric renal failure. The result is inability of the kidney to maintain water, electrolyte and acid-base homeostasis, or to eliminate waste products of metabolism.

257

Classification of the Degree of Renal Failure

Acute Tubular Necrosis

Potentially transient renal insult, which if promptly reversed by judicious fluid supplementation and/or low dose dopamine (5mcg/kg/min) may not progress to frank renal failure.

Acute Renal Failure

Compromise of renal function to the extent the following complications can develop:

Complication	Result
water retention	dilutional hyponatremia causing coma, seizures, lethargy
sodium retention	fluid overload causing: edema, hypertension, cardiac failure
Hyperkalemia	Cardiac rhythm and conduction disturbances
Metabolic acidosis	Impaired cellular metabolism
Uremic syndrome	accumulation of "uremic toxins" which eventually causes: anorexia, encephalopathy pericarditis, prolonged bleeding time

Dialysis may be required to support the patient until renal function has improved.

Chronic Renal Failure

In addition to the complications seen in acute renal failure, chronic renal failure is characterized by:

Malnutrition and growth failure. Dialysis can permit adequate calorie and protein intake to promote growth.

Renal osteodystrophy (Renal Rickets). In addition to added dietary Vitamin D and phosphate binders such as calcium carbonate, amelioration of this complication may require parathyroidectomy.

Anemia. An effective synthetic erythropoietin is now available which avoids the necessity of blood transfusions for this complication.

Hypertension. If present, treatment will be required to prevent additional insult to the kidney as well as other organs.

Hyperkalemia. Dietary potassium restriction is generally not needed until the GFR has decreased to less than 5 ml/min/1.73m^2.

May not require dialysis until the GFR has decreased to < 7-11 ml/min/1.73m^2.

End Stage Renal Disease

Treatment will require chronic dialysis (hemodialysis or peritoneal dialysis) or renal transplant.

Causes of Renal Failure

Prerenal

Decreased perfusion of the kidneys with resultant impaired substrate delivery to renal cells:

Hypotension

> Septicemia
> Cardiac failure
> Hemorrhage
> Neurogenic shock

Hypovolemia

> Hemorrhage
> Gastrointestinal fluid loss
> Hypoproteinemia
> Adrenal failure
> Burns

Severe hypertension

> Malignant hypertension

Hypoxemia

> Cardiac failure
> Respiratory failure
> Severe anemia

Hypoglycemia
Renal artery occlusion

Renal

Intrinsic renal parenchymal injury:

Glomerulonephritis

Poststreptococcal glomerulonephritis
Membranoproliferative glomerulonephritis
Lupus nephritis
Henoch-Schönlein purpura
Hereditary nephritis

Nephrotoxicity

Heavy metals
Nephrotoxic chemicals and drugs
Hemoglobin/myoglobin-uria
Shock
Acute tubular ischemia

Intravascular coagulation

Hemolytic-uremic syndrome
Disseminated intravascular coagulation
Cortical necrosis
Renal vein thrombosis

Developmental abnormalities

Cystic kidneys
Hypoplastic/dysplastic kidneys

Postrenal

Obstruction of urine flow from the kidneys:

Uric acid nephropathy
Lithiases
Extrinsic tumors
Vesicoureteral reflux
Structural abnormalities

Disease Profiles

Congenital Anomalies Associated with Renal Disease
Cystic Diseases
        Polycystic disease
                Autosomal recessive form (infantile)
                Autosomal dominant form (adult)
        Medullary cystic disease (Nephronophthisis)
                Autosomal recessive form (juvenile)
                Autosomal dominant form (Adult)
        Hereditary and familial cystic dysplasia
                Congenital nephrosis
                "Finnish" disease
Dysplastic Renal Diseases
        Renal aplasia
        Renal hypoplasia
        Multicystic renal dysplasia
        Familial and hereditary renal dysplasia
        Oligomeganephronia
Hereditary Diseases Associated with Nephritis
        Hereditary nephritis with deafness and ocular defects (Alport
          syndrome)
        Nail-patella syndrome
        Familial hyperprolinemia
        Hereditary nephrotic syndrome
        Hereditary osteolysis with nephropathy
        Hereditary nephritis with thoracic asphyxiant dystrophy syndrome
Hereditary Diseases Associated with Intrarenal Deposition of Metabolites
        Angiokeratome corporis diffusum (Fabry's disease)
        Heredopathia atatica polyneuritiformis (Refsum disease)
                Various storage diseases
                      G_{m1} monosialoganglilsidosis
                      Hurler syndrome
                      Niemann-Pick disease
                      Familial metachromatic leukodystrophy
                      Glycogenesis type I (von Gierke's disease)
                      Glycogenesis type II (Pompe's disease)

Hereditary amyloidosis
Familial Mediterranean fever
Heredofamilial urticaria with deafness and neuropathy
Primary familial amyloidosis with polyneuropathy
Hereditary Renal Diseases Associated With Tubular
  Transport Defects
    Hartnup disease
    Immunoglycinuria
    Fanconi's syndrome
    Oculocerebrorenal syndrome of Lowe
    Cystinosis
    Wilson's disease
    Galactosemia
    Hereditary fructose intolerance
    Renal tubular acidosis
    Hereditary tyrosinemia
    Renal glycosuria
    Vitamin D-resistant rickets
    Pseudohypoparathyroidism
    Vasopressin-resistant diabetes insipidus
    Hypouricemia
Hereditary Diseases Associated with Lithiasis
    Idiopathic hypercalciuria
    Hyperoxaluria
    L-Glyceric aciduria
    Xanthinuria
    Lesch-Nyhan syndrome
    Gout
    Familial hyperparathyroidism
    Cystinuria
    Glycinuria
Miscellaneous
    Hereditary intestinal vitamin B_{12} malabsorption
    Total and partial lipodystrophy
    Sickle cell anemia
    Bartter's syndrome

Modified from Gary M. Lum, MD, in *Current Pediatric Diagnosis and Treatment* (Hathaway, WE, et al editors), Appleton & Lange, 1991

Glomerular Disorders

Glomerular injury results in two distinct types of functional lesions: inflammatory and non-inflammatory. Non inflammatory glomerular lesions result in protein leakage through the injured filtering interface. These are referred to as nephrotic lesions. In uncomplicated cases, they do not compromise the GFR. Therefore, fluid retention, hypertension, and elevated BUN/Cr are not expected. The prototype of such lesions is seen in the idiopathic nephrotic syndrome of childhood. In inflammatory lesions (nephritic lesions) eroded areas allow loss of particles as large as RBCs, however, the swollen glomeruli decrease the total filtering surface available and cause fluid retention, hypertension and decreased GFR, as well as hematuria. Poststreptococcal glomerulonephritis is the protypical inflammatory glomerular lesion. Many glomerular disorders have components of both nephrotic and nephritic lesions.

Idiopathic Nephrotic Syndrome of Childhood
Most common cause of nephrotic syndrome in children
Alternate Terminology
Nil lesion nephrotic syndrome, minimal lesion nephrotic syndrome, lipoid nephrosis of childhood
Etiology
may be an abnormality of a thymic T-cell lymphocytic function resulting in increased permeability of glomerular filtering surfaces.
Pathophysiologic Abnormality
urinary protein loss > 40mg/M^2/hour
Predisposing Conditions
male (2:1), age 2-6 years, viral URI
Symptoms
anorexia, abdominal pain, diarrhea, lethargy
Physical Findings
edema
Laboratory Findings
proteinuria, hypoalbuminemia, hyperlipidemia, normal C3, BUN, Cr; no hematuria, or RBC casts
Chronologic Sequence of Manifestations
Proteinuria → hypoalbuminemia → edema (periorbital, then dependent, then generalized)

Potential Complications

Infections: peritonitis (*S. pneumoniae* most common) pneumonia, sepsis, cellulitis, UTI. Vascular thrombosis, steroid-induced cataracts

Differential Diagnosis

Focal segmental glomerulosclerosis, Mesangial proliferative glomerulonephritis

Diagnostic Plan

Urine: timed protein excretion, complete urinalysis Serum: BUN, Cr, electrolytes, C3, lipid profile, total protein/albumin

Therapeutic Plan

Prednisone 2mg/kg/day until proteinuria resolves or 4-6 weeks; then taper.

Prognosis

Good, if steroid responsive. 95% with minimal change disease respond to corticosteroids. If they do not, misdiagnosis must be considered. Relapses may occur with URIs and require retreatment.

Focal Segmental Glomerulosclerosis

Initially may be indistinguishable from minimal - change disease. Only 20% with this morphologic lesion respond to corticosteroids. The remainder progress to end stage renal disease, and, the disease recurs in transplanted kidneys.

Mesangial Proliferative Glomerulonephritis

Also called IgM Nephropathy

Has features of both minimal-change disease and focal segmental glomerulosclerosis. About 50% respond to corticosteroids, the others progress to end stage renal disease.

Hemolytic-Uremic Syndrome

Most common cause of acute renal failure in infants and children

Etiology

Has been associated with bacterial (especially *E coli* [O157:H7]), as well as viral gastrointestinal infections.

Pathophysiologic Abnormality

Renal vascular endothelial injury results from platelet deposition and consumption. Red cells are broken up as they pass through the fibrin strands, and renal perfusion is compromised. The result is the characteristic triad of azotemia, thrombocytopenia, and microangiopathic hemolytic anemia

Symptoms

fever, vomiting, diarrhea (often bloody), irritability, altered sensorium, oliguria

Physical Findings

edema, pallor, petechiae, hepatosplenomegaly

Laboratory Findings

Elevated BUN/Cr, anemia, elevated reticulocyte count, elevated bilirubin, leukocytosis, thrombocytopenia, negative Coombs' test, helmet/burr cells on peripheral smear, normal C3

Chronologic Sequence of Manifestations

gastroenteritis signs and symptoms followed by 7 to 10 days improvement, then acute onset of renal failure and anemia

Potential Complications

problems due to acute renal failure and diffuse vasculitis and/or intravascular thrombosis.

Differential Diagnosis

Bilateral renal vein thrombosis, lupus nephritis, acute glomerulonephritis

Therapeutic Plan

Treatment of the acute renal failure. Plasmapheresis is advocated by some.

Prognosis

Recovery of renal function has occurred after 2 or more weeks of anuria. Hypertension, chronic renal failure and CVAs or other intravascular thrombotic phenomena are worrisome potential late sequelae.

Poststreptococcal Glomerulonephritis

Competes with IgA nephropathy as the most common cause of gross hematuria in children

Etiology

Nephritogenic strains of group A beta- hemolytic streptococci

Pathophysiologic Abnormality
Inflammatory glomerular lesions causing decreased GFR and fluid retention

Predisposing Conditions
Streptococcal pharyngitis or impetigo

Symptoms
tea-colored urine, oliguria, lethargy, malaise,abdominal pain, flank pain, fever

Physical Findings
edema, hypertension, fluid overload

Laboratory Findings
urine: RBC casts, hematuria, proteinuria, WBCs.
serum: low C3 complement, positive Streptozyme test, elevated ASO titer (post pharyngitis; not impetigo), elevated BUN/Cr, normal proteins,

Chronologic Sequence of Manifestations
Streptococcal infection, then renal insult. The C3 returns to normal within 8 weeks

Potential Complications
renal failure with fluid overload, hypertension, uremia

Differential Diagnosis
other causes of hematuria

Diagnostic Plan
monitor BP, urinalysis, C3 complement, BUN/Cr, CBC, Streptozyme test, Protein

Therapeutic Plan
sodium and fluid restriction, loop diuretics, antihypertensives, if BP elevated

Prognosis
95% recover completely. Morbidity may result from uncontrolled hypertension.

Postinfectious Non-Streptococcal Glomerulonephritis
Other causes of acute infection-mediated glomerulonephritis include:
Bacterial: staphylococcal (shunt nephritis); Viral: hepatitis B, infectious mononucleosis, CMV infections; Fungal: histoplasmosis; Parasitic: toxoplasmosis, falciparum malaria

Membranoproliferative Glomerulonephritis
Most common cause of chronic glomerulonephritis in older children and adults.
Also called mesangiocapillary GMN. Once differentiated from other causes of chronic GMN by the finding of decreased C3, but now distinguished by 3 histologic subtypes:
Type I
Type II
Type III
Presents in the 2nd decade of life with proteinuria and hematuria. Most develop nephrotic syndrome. Many progress to end stage renal disease. Renal biopsy is required for the diagnosis since hypocomplementemia does not always occur.

Membranous Glomerulopathy
Most common cause of nephrotic syndrome in adults
Clinical manifestations are similar to membranoproliferative GMN except the C3 is normal, and most cases in children resolve spontaneously.

Rapidly Progressive Glomerulonephritis
Also called diffuse crescentic GMN. If the typical glomerular crescents are not due to poststreptococcal, membranoproliferative, anaphylactoid purpura, lupus or Goodpasture disease progression to end stage renal disease can be expected within months of onset. C3 is normal. Diagnosis is made by renal biopsy.

Hereditary Glomerulonephritis
The most common form is Alport's syndrome which presents around school age with asymptomatic hematuria followed by development of proteinuria. Many have hypertension, which may be severe, and one-third have sensorineural hearing loss. Eye problems also occur in 15% of patients.

Lupus Nephritis
Nephritis is a common manifestation of lupus erythematosus in childhood. Adolescent females are most commonly affected. Normalization of C3 reflects effective immunosuppressive therapy. The renal injury may progress to end stage renal disease. It is a disease characterized by remissions and relapses as it progresses. Complications may occur both from the disease and from the therapy it requires.

IgA Nephropathy
   Alternate Terminology
      Berger's nephropathy
   Pathogenesis
      IgA deposition on glomerular basement membranes
   Predisposing Conditions
      URIs, male sex
   Laboratory Findings
      Normal C3, microscopic and gross hematuria, non-nephrotic proteinuria
   Potential Complications
      20% develop hypertension, nephrotic syndrome, and eventual renal failure. The nephropathy recurs in transplanted kidneys.

Henoch-Schönlein Purpura Glomerulonephritis
   Alternate Terminology
      Anaphylactoid purpura GMN
   Pathophysiologic Abnormality
      Small vessel vasculitis, which can cause decreased GFR
   Symptoms
      abdominal pain, arthralgia
   Physical Findings
      urticarial and/or purpuric rash on buttocks and lower extremities, joint effusions
   Laboratory Findings
      hematuria, proteinuria, normal C3 and platelets
   Chronologic Sequence of Manifestations
      Urticarial rash progresses to palpable purpuric lesions. Abdominal pain which promptly resolves following institution of corticosteroid therapy is typical
   Potential Complications
      Intussusception, bowel perforation. Severe renal involvement is rare.
   Prognosis
      When severe renal involvement occurs, it is unresponsive to treatment.

Sickle Cell Nephropathy

The initial defect is usually in concentrating ability of the tubules. Renal involvement may progress to include episodic hematuria and a nephrotic syndrome.

Juxtaglomerular Disorders

Histologically demonstrable juxtaglomerular disorders are extremely rare, but the disorders in its differential are not. Urine chloride is helpful since those disorders associated with hypovolemia have low urine chloride levels.

Bartter Syndrome
Pathology
Generalized hyperplasia of the juxtaglomerular apparatus
Pathophysiologic Abnormality
A defect in chloride reabsorption in the ascending loop of Henle results in urinary potassium wasting when excess NaCl presents to the distal tubule and is reabsorbed in exchange for potassium. Hypokalemia stimulates prostaglandin and renin synthesis. The elevated prostaglandin contributes to a defect in platelet aggregation, and the elevated renin stimulates aldosterone production which exacerbates the hypokalemia.
Symptoms
muscle weakness, polyuria, constipation, carpo-pedal spasms
Physical Findings
dehydration, growth failure, normal blood pressure
Laboratory Findings
severe hypokalemia, defective platelet aggregation, hypochloremic metabolic alkalosis, elevated renin, elevated aldosterone, elevated prostaglandin E_2, elevated urine potassium, elevated urine chloride.
Differential Diagnosis
licorice abuse, pyelonephritis, diabetes insipidus, chronic vomiting, chronic diarrhea, laxative abuse, diuretic use

Interstitial Disorders

Acute Interstitial Nephritis
A disorder of unknown etiology characterized by interstitial inflammation and edema. Most often due to drug therapy and in such cases may be a hypersensitivity reaction. It is also seen in association with infections and other disorders, including renal transplant rejection. Staining of the urinary sediment for eosinophils may be helpful in identifying this entity. Diagnosis is made by renal biopsy.

Chronic Interstitial Nephritis
Once the interstitial edema of acute interstitial nephritis is replaced by fibrosis, the condition is progressive and end-stage renal failure ensues.

Tubular Disorders

Renal Tubular Acidosis
A heterogeneous group of disorders, all of which have hyperchloremic metabolic acidosis, and tubular dysfunction. Renal failure is not an expected component of this group of disorders.

Renal Tubular Acidosis Type I
Alternate Terminology
   Distal renal tubular acidosis
Etiology
   May be primary or secondary to obstructive uropathy, pyelonephritis, sickle cell nephropathy, lupus nephritis, medullary sponge kidney, renal transplant rejection, or toxins
Pathophysiologic Abnormality
   Defective hydrogen ion secretion in the distal tubule, which results in up to 15% of the filtered sodium bicarbonate load being lost in the urine.
Symptoms
   failure to thrive, anorexia, vomiting
Physical Findings
   dehydration

Laboratory Findings
> hyperchloremic metabolic acidosis, mild hypokalemia, alkaline urine

Potential Complications
> hypercalciuria, nephrocalcinosis, renal stones

Therapeutic Plan
> 2-3 mEq/kg/24hr $NaHCO_3$ is therapeutic and distinguishes this from the proximal type which requires > 10 mEq/kg/24hr.

Prognosis
> good if renal injury can be avoided

Renal Tubular Acidosis Type II

Alternate Terminology
> Proximal renal tubular acidosis

Etiology
> May be primary, a component of Fanconi syndrome, or due to tubular immaturity in premature infants

Pathophysiologic Abnormality
> Lowered renal threshold for bicarbonate reabsorption in the proximal tubule. If serum acidosis drops below this threshold, the urine becomes acidic.

Laboratory Findings
> hyperchloremic metabolic acidosis, hypokalemia

Potential Complications
> rarely nephrocalcinosis

Therapeutic Plan
> high (> 5 mEq/kg/24hr) doses of bicarbonate

Prognosis
> Excellent if isolated lesion, otherwise dependent on underlying disorder.

Renal Tubular Acidosis Type III

Type I with an associated bicarbonate tubular leak

Renal Tubular Acidosis Type IV

Alternate Terminology
> Mineralocorticoid deficiency RTA

Etiology

Disorders with:

decreased aldosterone and elevated renin: Adrenal failure, Congenital adrenal hyperplasia, Primary hypoaldosteronism

decreased aldosterone and decreased renin: pyelonephritis, interstitial nephritis, obstructive lesions, nephrosclerosis, diabetes mellitus

increased aldosterone and increased renin: Pseudohypoaldosteronism

Diffuse Proximal Renal Tubular Dysfunction

Alternate Terminology

Fanconi syndrome

Etiology

Inherited disorders: Cystinosis, Lowe syndrome, Galactosemia, Tyrosinemia, Hereditary fructose intolerance, Glycogen storage disease type I, Wilson disease, Medullary cystic disease Systemic disorders: Rubella syndrome, Amyloidosis, Sjögren syndrome Toxins: heavy metals, outdated tetracycline, Lindane, hyperparathyroidism, interstitial nephritis

Pathophysiologic Abnormality

Defect in proximal tubular function

Laboratory Findings

Hyperchloremic metabolic acidosis, glycosuria, aminoaciduria, depressed tubular reabsorption of phosphate

Prognosis

Dependent on the underlying disorder

Nephrogenic Diabetes Insipidus

Etiology

Primary form is X-linked recessive and completely expressed and only partly in females. All forms are diagnosed by lack of response to vasopressin.

Urologic Disorders

If the following are considered possibilities in the differential diagnosis of causes of azotemia in children, imaging studies may be indicated.

Hydronephrosis

Urolithiasis

Neurogenic bladder

Urethral stenosis

Posterior urethral valves

> Should always be considered in the differential of causes of azotemia in male infants.

Hypospadias

> Avoid circumcisions, since the foreskin is used in repair of the lesion.

Cryptorchidism

> Should be surgically corrected (orchiopexy) by age 2 years.

Testicular torsion

> A true surgical emergency as delayed correction can lead to loss of the testicle.

A Eugene Osburn

Developmental Considerations

Fluid Spaces

Total Body Water

70-75% of total body weight in the newborn. After the postnatal diuresis, it is 65% and remains constant until puberty when it decreases to 55-60%. About 2/3 of the TBW is intracellular and the rest extracellular fluid.

Extracellular Fluid

Sodium is the predominant cation of the ECF. It is present in a concentration of 140 mEq/L. ECF contains only 4 mEq/L of potassium. Regulation of the ECF volume is through the interaction of the antidiuretic hormone (ADH), thirst and the renin-angiotensin-aldosterone axis. Distribution of fluid between the two compartments of the ECF (**Plasma Fluid** and **Interstitial Fluid**) is regulated primarily by the oncotic pressure of plasma proteins. The clinical signs of dehydration are a reflection of changes in the ECF volume.

Intracellular Fluid

Potassium is the major cation in the ICF. Its concentration there is around 160 mEq/L.

Diagnostic Modalities

Osmolality

This is the mechanism which governs distribution of body fluids across the compartments' semipermeable membranes. The normal osmolality is 285 mosm/L.

Osmolar Gap

The difference between measured osmolality and calculated osmolality. The expected osmolality can be calculated by the formula:

$$\text{Plasma osmolality} = 2 \times (Na^+) + \frac{\text{Glucose}}{18} + \frac{\text{BUN}}{2.8}$$

Causes of Abnormal Saline Concentrations

Sodium imbalance may be due to an excess or deficit of either the sodium or the water containing it. As a first step, it is helpful to determine whether the imbalance is accompanied by dehydration (ie, decreased total body water) or whether the imbalance exists with normal or excessive total body water.

The most accurate way to determine whether total body water is decreased, normal or increased is by recent weight changes in the child, though this information is often not available. If edema is present, there is an increase in both sodium and total body water. Whether the child is hypernatremic, hyponatremic or has a sodium in the normal range merely reflects the concentration of sodium, not the total amount present. In children with healthy kidneys, the urine sodium reflects a regulatory response to excess or depletion of total body sodium, as well as to total body water. Thus if there is a total body deficit of sodium, the urine sodium concentration will be low whether the child's serum sodium concentration reflects hypernatremia or hyponatremia.

A second mechanism involved is maintaining vascular perfusion is the antidiuretic hormone (ADH) action on distal tubes. In addition to causing an elevation in mean arterial pressure due to arteriolar vasoconstriction, this hormone's effect may be perpetuate or worsen hyponatremia if the child has severe enough vascular volume depletion. Vascular volume will be maintained to the extent it can via the release of ADH even if doing so results in hyponatremia in the extracellular fluid.

The clinical assessment of dehydration is based on parameters which reflect reduction in extracellular fluid and vascular volume. Remember that fluid shifts into or out-of the intracellular fluid space will alter the amount of total body water loss required to cause the findings associated with clinical mild, moderate or severe dehydration. Hyponatremia is associated with a shift of fluids into the cells and thus the clinical signs of degree of dehydration will occur with less fluid loss. The converse is true in hypernatremia dehydration. By the time clinically severe dehydration, based on clinical findings, occurs in patients with hypernatremic dehydration, the child is in danger of catastrophic vascular collapse because of the amount of total body water lost.

Clinical Assessment of Degree of Dehydration			
Parameter			
	Mild (< 5%)	**Moderate (10%)**	**Severe (15%)**
Skin Color	Pink	Acrocyanosis	Mottled
Tears	Present	Reduced	Absent
Mucous Membrane	Normal	Dry	Parched
Eyeball	Normal	Depressed	Sunken
Fontanelle	Normal	Depressed	Sunken
Level of Consciousness	Alert	Lethargic	Obtunded
Pulse Rate	Upper Normal	Increased	Markedly Increased
Capillary Refill	Upper Normal	Definitely Prolonged	Markedly Prolonged
Blood Pressure	Normal	Orthostatic Hypotension	Recumbent Hypotension
BUN	Normal	Elevated	Very High
Arterial pH	7.40 - 7.30	7.30 - 7.00	< 7.10
Urine			
Volume	Small	Oliguria	Oliguria/anuria
Specific Gravity	< 1.020	> 1.030	> 1.035

Causes of Hypernatremia
    Hypernatremia Associated with Decreased ECF
        due to extrarenal water losses (urine $Na < 10$ mEq/L)
            skin losses
            respiratory losses
            gastrointestinal losses
            severe burns
            thyrotoxicosis
        due to renal water losses (urine $Na > 40$ mEq/L)
            diuretics
            renal disease
            relief of urinary obstruction
            osmoreceptor failure

Hypernatremia Associated with Normal ECF
impaired thirst
nonrenal water losses
renal water losses

Hypernatremia associated with increased ECF
iatrogenic saline excess
mineralocorticoid excess
      hyperaldosteronism
      Cushings disease
      exogenous corticosteroid

Causes of Hyponatremia

Hyponatremia Associated with Decreased ECF
due to extrarenal sodium losses (urine Na < 20 mEq/L)
    sweating
    vomiting/diarrhea
    burn fluid loss
    peritonitis
    pancreatitis
due to renal sodium losses (urine Na > 40 mEq/L)
    aldosterone deficiency
    congenital adrenal hyperplasia
    salt losing nephropathy
    renal tubular diuretics
    osmotic diuretics

Hyponatremia associated with normal ECF
[Normal BUN, no edema]
    inappropriate ADH secretion (SIADH)
    "appropriate" excess ADH secretion
        pain, physical/emotional stress
        myxedema
    without excess ADH secretion
        water intoxication
            iatrogenic water overload
            psychogenic polydipsia
    Sick cell (reset osmostat) syndrome

Hyponatremia Associated with Increased ECF
  decreased GFR and abnormal tubules (oliguria, urine sodium > 40 mEq/L)
    renal failure
  decreased GFR with normal tubules (oliguria, urine sodium < 20 mEq/L)
    [decreased vascular volume and/or cardiac output]
    cardiac failure
    hepatic failure
    nephrotic syndrome
Factitious Hyponatremia
  hyperglycemia
  hyperlipidemia
  hyperproteinemia

Since glucose remains extracellular in hyperglycemia, it draws intracellular water into the extracellular space and factitiously dilutes the measured sodium there. The true serum sodium concentration in hyperglycemia can be calculated by assuming the sodium is diluted 1.6 to 1.8 mEq/L for each 100 mg/dl the glucose is above its normal 100 mg/dl.

Fluid and Electrolyte Treatment Guidelines

Daily Fluid Requirements	
Body Weight (kg)	**Maintenance Water Required**
Up to 10	100 cc/kg
11-20	1000 cc + 50 cc/kg for each kg over 10 kg
Above 20	1500 cc/kg + 20 cc/kg for each kg over 20 kg

Daily Electrolyte Requirements	
Cation	**Maintenance Requirements**
Sodium	3 mEq/kg/24 hours
Potassium	2 mEq/kg/24 hours

Maintenance Fluids

Maintenance fluids can be provided by using D_5W 1/4 NS plus 20-30 mEq/L KCl. The infusion rate can be calculated using the expected 24 hour fluid volume requirement guidelines given above, or can be directly calculated as an hourly rate by the following:

Hourly Maintenance Fluid Rate

0 to 10 kg:	4 cc/kg/hr
11 to 20 kg:	40 cc/hr + 2 cc/kg/hr for each kg > 10
> 20 kg:	60 cc/kg/hr + 1 cc/kg/hr for each kg > 20

Treatment of Electrolyte Imbalances

Hypernatremia

Hypernatremia with edema and a normal BUN (unless in shock) is due to salt poisoning and requires urgent dialysis.

The serum sodium in hypernatremic dehydration must be replaced slowly, over 48 hours, to avoid too rapid osmolar shifts of water into brain cells with resulting cerebral edema. For the same reason, the replacement fluid should be at least 1/4 Normal Saline, not dextrose in water alone.

The degree of dehydration estimated from clinical signs of dehydration relies on findings reflecting the extracellular fluid volume. In hypernatremic dehydration the amount of fluid loss is often underestimated because the fluid shift from the intracellular space in hypertonic dehydration delays clinical manifestations of the amount of TBW lost. The actual water deficit in hypernatremic dehydration can be estimated by:

Normal total body water (TBW) = 0.6 X normal wt (kg)

$$\frac{\text{Normal Na}}{\text{Measured Na}} \quad X \quad TBW \quad = \quad \text{current TBW}$$

Fluid deficit = Normal TBW - current TBW

Hyponatremia

Symptomatic hyponatremia rarely occurs unless the serum Na is less than 120 mEq/L, and symptoms such as seizures are more the result of the rapidity of fall in sodium concentration than the level reached.

A key to assessing the approach to treatment of hyponatremia is the BUN.

Hyponatremia with a normal BUN is due either to inappropriate ADH secretion or water intoxication and the treatment of either of these conditions is water restriction, not fluid replacement, unless the hyponatremia is symptomatic.

Symptomatic hyponatremia may be treated with hypertonic saline (3%). The volume required to raise the serum Na above 120 mEq/L can be calculated by the formula:

(Desired Na [ie, 120 mEq/L] - measured Na) X 0.6 X wt (kg) = mEq Na required.

3% saline contains 0.5 mEq Na/cc.

Symptomatic hyponatremia will usually respond to raising the serum sodium concentration 10 mEq/L; correction of the remainder of the imbalance should be done more slowly.

Hyperkalemia

Physiologically significant hyperkalemia is reflected in the EKG. The earliest change in the EKG is a tenting or peaking of the T waves.

Treatment of hyperkalemia includes calcium gluconate (calcium chloride can worsen acidosis usually present in hyperkalemic conditions), sodium bicarbonate, insulin and glucose, and a cation exchange resin (Kayexalate). These are listed in descending order of rapidity on onset of action and ascending order of duration of action. Dialysis may be needed for situations not adequately controlled by the preceding temporary measures.

Hypokalemia

Total body potassium deficits are not necessarily reflected in serum potassium values. A urine potassium of < 20 mEq/L, however, reflects the normal kidney's effort to conserve the potassium presented to its tubules.

Thus, urine potassium should guide replacement of total body potassium deficits.

Physiologically significant hypokalemia is reflected in the EKG with ST segment depression, T wave amplitude reduction and U waves.

Except in unusual circumstances, potassium concentration in IV fluids should not exceed 40 mEq/L.

Guidelines for Treatment of Dehydration						
	Weight Loss per Severity			Replacement Fluid	Hours for Deficit Replacement	
	Mild	Moderate	Severe		1st 1/2	2nd 1/2
Hypotonic dehydration	2%	5%	10%	D_5W 3/4 NS	4	20
Isotonic dehydration	5%	10%	15%	D_5W 1/2 NS	8	16
Hypertonic dehydration	10%	15%	20%	D_5W 1/4 NS	24	24

1. Correct shock with boluses of 20 cc/kg of D_5W NS. If additional volume is needed use plasminate or albumin.
2. Obtain results for BUN, Cr, Na, K, Cl, HCO, and glucose
3. Estimate severity of dehydration.
4. Based on severity estimated and type identified with the electrolyte results, multiply the percent from the above by body weight and using the composition of fluid from the replacement fluid column replace one half the deficit volume over each of the number of hours depicted.
5. Add KCl in a concentration of 20 - 40 mEq/L to the replacement fluid as soon as adequate urine flow is assured.

The above volumes and concentrations should be added to the daily maintenance fluid requirement to avoid getting behind from failing to provide ongoing needs.

Therapeutic Endpoints for Treatment of Dehydration	
Goal	**Time Frame**
Adequate urine volume	First hour
Urine specific gravity = 1.010	First few hours*
Normal electrolytes	Hours (hyponatremia) to 2 days (hyperatremia)
Elevated BUN decreased by 1/2	Every 15 - 20 hours
Normal Acid-Base Status	One to three days
Urine potassium > 40 mEq/L	Three to five days

* After the urine specific gravity has decreased to 1.010, the infusion rate of fluids can be decreased to maintenance rates since the kidneys will just excrete any excess at that point.

Acid-Base Disturbances

A pH of 7.40 is the result of a ratio of HCO_3 to $PaCO_2$ of 20 to 1. Changes in this ratio cause a corresponding change in the pH. This is reflected in the following formula:

$$pH = \frac{HCO_3}{PaCO_2} = \frac{24 \text{ mEq/L}}{40 \text{ mm Hg}} = \frac{20}{1} = 7.40$$

$$(40 \text{ mm Hg} \times 0.03 = 1.2 \text{ mEq/L})$$

The $PaCO_2$ is dependent on the minute volume of respiration and can change in minutes. The HCO_3 is regulated by the kidneys and changes take hours to days. Any change in either of these determiners of pH is accompanied by a compensatory change in the other. The results of such changes is depicted in the table that follows:

	HCO$_3$ mEq/L < 21	HCO$_3$ mEq/L 21 -26	HCO$_3$ mEq/L > 26
PaCo$_2$ mm Hg > 45	Combined Metabolic Acidosis and Respiratory Acidosis	Respiratory Acidosis	Mixed Metabolic Alkalosis and Respiratory Acidosis
PaCO$_2$ mm Hg 35-45	Metabolic Acidosis	**NORMAL**	Metabolic Alkalosis
PaCo$_2$ mm Hg < 35	Mixed Metabolic Acidosis and Respiratory Alkalosis	Respiratory Alkalosis	Combined Respiratory Alkalosis and Metabolic Alkalosis

In mixed disorders, the pH reflects which mixed disorder pair is primary and which is secondary since compensation is never complete nor over-compensated. The mechanisms for the compensatory changes are:

Expected Compensatory Changes in Primary Acid-Base Disorders

Disorder	Initial Change	Compensatory Change
Respiratory Acidosis	10 mm Hg $PaCO_2$ increase	HCO_3 increases 1 mEq/L (acute) HCO_3 increases 3-4 mEq/L (chronic)
Respiratory Alkalosis	10 mm Hg $PaCO_2$ decrease	HCO_3 decreases 1-3 mEq/L (acute) HCO_3 decreases 2-5 mEq/L (chronic)
Metabolic Acidosis	1 mEq/L HCO_3 decrease	$PaCO_2$ decreases 1-1.5 mm Hg
Metabolic Alkalosis	1 mEq/L HCO_3 increase	$PaCO_2$ increases 0.5-1 mm Hg

---

General Acid-Base Rules of Thumb

A 1 mm Hg increase in $PaCo_2$ causes a 0.01 decrease in pH.

A 1 mEq/L decrease in HCO_3 causes a 0.02 decrease in pH.

A 0.1 increase in pH causes a 0.5 mEq/L decrease in K+.

A 0.1 increase in pH shifts the oxygen dissociation curve to the left enough to decrease O_2 release to tissues by 10%.

In primary metabolic acidosis, the $PaCO_2$ in mm Hg should equal the 2 digits to the right of the decimal point of the pH if no other derangement exists. eg, a pH of 7.22 corresponds to a $PaCO_2$ of 22 mm Hg in pure acute metabolic acidosis without compensatory changes.

Causes of Metabolic Alkalosis

Chloride Responsive Causes (urine Cl < 10 mEq/L)

gastrointestinal chloride loss

vomiting

gastric suction

chloride diarrhea

diuretics
rapid correction of hypercapnia
Cystic Fibrosis
Chloride-Resistant Causes (urine Cl > 20 mEq/L)
excess mineralocorticoid activity
hyperaldosteronism
Cushings syndrome
Bartters syndrome
excess licorice
severe K depletion
Variable Chloride Response
Milk-alkali syndrome
alkali administration

Causes of Metabolic Acidosis
Increased Loss of Bicarbonate or Chloride Addition (normal anion gap)
associated with potassium retention (hyperkalemia)
early uremic acidosis
renal tubular acidosis type IV
hyopaldosteronism
potassium sparing diuretics
resolving DKA
early obstructive uropathy
associated with potassium depletion (hypokalemia)
acute diarrhea with HCO and Cl losses
renal tubular acidosis type I
renal tubular acidosis type II
dilution acidosis
Increased Organic Acids (increased anion gap)
A   aspirin, alcohol ketoacidosis
M   methanol
U   uremia
D   diabetic ketoacidosis
P   paraldehyde
I   iron, ibuprofen, isoniazid
L   lactic acidosis
E   ethylene glycol
S   starvation ketoacidosis

Anion Gap

The anion gap reflects the amount of organic acids present in the serum. It can be calculated by the formula:

$$\text{Anion gap} = (Na^+ + K^+) - (Cl^- + HCO_3^-) = 8 \text{ to } 12 \text{ mEq/L}$$

Causes of Respiratory Alkalosis

Anxiety/Hyperventilation

CNS Pathology

infection, trauma, tumors

Hypoxia

mild bronchospasm

congestive heart failure

pneumonia

pulmonary emboli

severe anemia

Respiratory Center Stimulating Drugs

salicylates

catecholamines

Pregnancy

Pain

Fever/sepsis

Hepatic dysfunction

Hyperthyroidism

Causes of Respiratory Acidosis

CNS Depression of Respiratory Drive

drug overdose

CNS lesions

CNS infections

Pulmonary Diseases

obstructive pulmonary disease

severe bronchospasm

pneumonia

pulmonary edema

smoke inhalation

Mechanical Abnormalities
  airway obstruction
  foreign body
  croup
  epiglottitis
  retropharyngeal abscess
  laryngeal edema
  aspiration
  pleural effusion
  pneumothorax
  flail chest
  scoliosis

Neuromuscular Abnormalities
  Guillain-Barré syndrome
  poliomyelitis
  Wernig-Hoffman disease
  myasthenia gravis
  botulism
  tetanus
  muscular dystrophy
  severe hypokalemia
  myxedema

A Eugene Osburn

Developmental Considerations

Optimal brain growth and development requires structural integrity, adequate nutritional substrates at the appropriate time, absence of toxic and traumatic insults and environmental stimulation. Deficiencies in any of these areas can result in suboptimal neurological development.

The skull grows in response to developing brain tissue. Microcephaly is due to smaller than average brain volume. Lack of skull growth does not cause microcephaly.

Physical brain growth continues until around ten years of age. At birth, the head is nearly 2/3 the adult size. More than 8/10 the adult size is reached by one year of age. Myelinization of the spinal cord is not completed until two years after birth.

Diagnostic Modalities

Serum Electrolytes, Glucose, Magnesium and Calcium
A fingerstick glucose should be done early in evaluation of altered sensorium. Hypoglycemia can cause profound and (if not rapidly enough reversed) permanent CNS changes. Determination of the other electrolytes and minerals may detect treatable causes of CNS dysfunction.

Toxicology Screens
A toxicology screen should always be considered in cases in which neurologic changes do not have an obvious explanation. In seizure patients with neurologic changes anticonvulsant levels are indicated.

Lumbar Puncture (LP) and Cerebrospinal Fluid (CSF) Analysis
The most common parameters assessed via a LP are: opening pressure, CSF cell count, CSF protein, CSF glucose, Counter Current Immune Electrophoresis (CCIE), and Gram stain. In uncooperative infants and children, the opening pressure may not be done because of questionable validity. Before performing the LP, one must be sure there is no evidence of significant increased intracranial pressure by noting the absence of papilledema, or, if time and the situation permit and indicate, a CT scan of the head. Focal neurologic deficits should especially raise the question of significant intracranial mass effect.

				Cells		
Age	Opening Pressure	Glucose	Protein	Polys	Lymphs	RBCs
Newborn	70 - 180 mm H$_2$O	50 -80 mg/dl	150 mg/dl	< 8	< 30	< 50
3 months		(2/3 of blood glucose)	< 65 mg/dl	< 3	< 15	< 30
> 6 months	70 - 150		10 - 40 mg/dl	0	< 5	< 5

*(Table title: **Normal CSF Values**)*

Electroencephalography (EEG)

The electroencephalogram is being replaced by MRI, evoked potentials, CT scans, and regional blood flow studies as both a diagnostic and prognostic tool in many of the neurological conditions. It was relied on before the availability of these modalities. It is still useful to confirm, classify the type of seizure, and monitor response to anticonvulsant therapy in seizure disorders.

Evoked Potentials

Computer enhanced averaging of responses to cortical auditory, visual, or somatosensory-evoked responses can be used by skilled interpreters to arrive at clinical interpretations of brain functional integrity with fairly reproducible results. They are becoming an extremely useful adjunct to the neurologic exam.

CT Scan of the Head

The CT scan can reveal structural abnormalities, midline shifts from mass lesions, acute and chronic bleeds, tumors and cerebral edema.

A CT without contrast media is indicated in suspected acute CNS bleeds. It may not, however, detect chronic subdural hematomas if the clot has organized sufficiently to be of similar density to surrounding brain tissue.

A CT with contrast media is needed to best delineate vascularized tumors, A-V malformations and chronic subdural clots. Contrast media should not be used if the patient has evidence of decreased GFR (elevated BUN/Cr), as its use in that situation can result in renal shutdown.

Magnetic Resonance Imaging (MRI)

The MRI is a noninvasive technique that provides more detailed delineation of white and gray matter of the brain and can provide information about not only structural abnormalities, but histological and biochemical information as well. It cannot detect calcified lesions, however, and it requires much longer immobilization. It usually requires sedation in children.

Pathophysiologic Manifestations

Common Causes of Altered Mental Status in Children By Age Group

Infant
Birth asphyxia
Infection
Inborn Error of Metabolism
Abuse
Metabolic Disorders

Child
Ingestion
Infection
Intussusception
Seizure
Abuse

Adolescent
Ingestion
Intentional
Trauma
Drug/Alcohol Abuse

Causes of Seizures By Age Group

First Day of Life
Hypoxia
Drugs
Trauma
Infection

Hyperglycemia
Hypoglycemia
Pyridoxine Deficiency

Days 2-3 of Life
Infection
Drug Withdrawal
Hypoglycemia
Hypocalcemia

Developmental Malformation
Intracranial Hemorrhage
Inborn Error of Metabolism
Hyponatremia/Hypernatremia

One Week to Six Months of Life
Infection
Hypocalcemia
Hyperphosphatemia
Hyponatremia

Developmental Malformation
Drug Withdrawal
Inborn Error of Metabolism

Six Months to 3 Years of Age
Febrile Seizures
Birth Injury
Infection
Toxins

Trauma
Metabolic Disorder
Cerebral Degenerative Disease

Over 3 Years of Age
Idiopathic
Infection

Trauma
Cerebral Degenerative Disease

Differentiating Upper Motor Neuron from Lower Motor Unit Lesions

Finding	Upper Motor Neuron	Motor Unit
Posture	Arm flexed, leg extended	Flaccid
Reflexes	Increased	Decreased or absent
Tone	Increased	Decreased
Fasciculations	Absent	Present
Atrophy	Absent or minimal	Present
Muscles Affected	Muscle groups	Individual muscles or groups

Upper motor neuron: the corticospinal tract and its motor neurons
Motor unit: includes lower motor neuron (the anterior horn cells, motor nerves, and peripheral motor nerves), neuromuscular junction and muscles.

Diseases of the Lower Motor Unit in Infants and Children

Anterior Horn Cell
  Spinal muscular atrophy (Werding-Hoffmann disease)
  Poliomyelitis
Peripheral Nerve
  Guillain-Barré syndrome
  Tick paralysis
Neuromuscular Junction
  Myasthenia gravis
  Botulism
Muscle
  Muscular Dystrophy
    Duchenne
    Becker
    Limb girdle
    Fascioscapulohumeral
    Myotonic
    Congenital
Metabolic, Endocrine, and Mineral
  Glycogen Storage disease type II (Pompe disease)
  Carnitine Metabolism abnormalities
  Mitochondrial abnormalities
  Thyroid excess or deficiency
  Cortisol excess or deficiency
  Hyperparathyroidism; calcium excess
  Potassium excess or deficiency

Disease Profiles

Disorders of embryogenesis (occur during first 4 weeks of gestation):

Neural Tube Defects
> **Alternate Terminology**
>> Posterior midline lesions
>> Dysraphia
>
> **Etiology**
>> Failure of neural groove to fuse completely during formation of the neural tube.
>
> **Pathophysiologic Abnormality**
>> Anencephaly - failure of brain to develop
>> Spina Bifida Cystica
>> Meningocele - herniation of the meninges
>> Meningomyelocele - herniation of the meninges and spinal cord
>> Arnold-Chiari Malformation - elongation and protrusion through the foramen magnum of medullary and cerebellar tissue
>> Tethered Cord - prevents upward migration of the spinal cord
>> Diplomyelia - duplication of spinal cord
>> Diastematomyelia - cleft in spinal cord
>> Syringomyelia - fluid-filled cyst in the spinal cord
>> Sacral Dysgenesis - seen in 1% of infants of diabetic mothers
>> Neurodermal Sinus - may be a site of entry for recurrent CNS infections
>> Spina Bifida Occulta - clinically benign defect of posterior aspect of vertebral bodies in lower lumbar area.
>
> **Clinical Findings and Prognosis**
>> Depend on level and severity of lesions

Disorders of cellular proliferation and migration:

Agenesis of Corpus Callosum
> **Pathophysiologic Abnormality**
>> Ventricles are farther apart than normal on CT
>
> **Predisposing Conditions**
>> Maternal ingestion of toxic substances, genetic abnormalities

Symptoms

Seizure disorder, severe retardation or no symptoms at all

Prognosis

Depends on severity

Microcephaly

Pathophysiologic Abnormality

Head circumference is more than 2 standard deviations below the norm

Predisposing Conditions

Chromosomal anomaly, idiopathic, hypothyroidism, Hurler syndrome, rickets, craniosynostosis

Macrocephaly

Etiology

Hydrocephalus is most common cause in infants. Inherited metabolic anomalies, chromosomal anomalies, arachnoid cysts, leukodystrophies.

Hydrancephaly

Etiology

Necrosis of cerebral cortex in utero

Prognosis

Usually die within first year of life

Hydrocephalus

Alternate Terminology

Types:

Noncommunicating hydrocephalus - due to obstruction of CSF flow

Communicating hydrocephalus - due to abnormal absorption of CSF

Pathophysiologic Abnormality

Enlargement of cerebral ventricles due to accumulation of CSF

Predisposing Conditions

Prenatal, perinatal - intraventricular bleeds, infections or malformations

Postnatal - brain tumors are most common cause

Symptoms

Accelerated rate of head growth, irritability, headaches, vomiting

Diagnostic Plan

Head CT

Therapeutic Plan

May require shunting

Cerebellar malformations:

Dandy-Walker Malformation
> **Pathophysiologic Abnormality**
>> Cystic dilation of the fourth ventricle with resulting hydrocephalus
>
> **Predisposing Conditions**
>> Atresia or blockage of the foramen of Magendie and foramen of Luschka
>
> **Prognosis**
>> Shunting is always required

Neurocutaneous syndromes - affects brain, skin and eyes; most inherited:

Neurofibromatosis
> **Alternate Terminology**
>> von Recklinghausen's disease
>
> **Etiology**
>> Autosomal dominant inheritance
>
> **Physical Findings**
>> 6 or more café au lait spots are diagnostic; neurofibromasi Lisch nodules - pigmented nodules in iris are present in 90% of patients
>
> **Potential Complications**
>> Optic nerve gliomas, acoustic neuromas, meningiomas, spinal cord tumors
>
> **Therapeutic Plan**
>> Genetic counseling is warranted

Tuberous Sclerosis
> **Alternate Terminology**
>> Bournville's disease
>
> **Etiology**
>> Autosomal dominant inheritance
>
> **Pathophysiologic Abnormality**
>> Triad of skin lesions, seizures, mental retardation
>
> **Symptoms**
>> Epilepsy, mental retardation, autistic features
>
> **Physical Findings**
>> Ash-leaf spots seen with Woods lamp, shagreen patches, café au lait spots, angiokeriotomas on face during second decade of life. Retinal hamartomas in 50% of patients

Potential Complications

Periventricular tumors, cysts and malignant tumors in the heart, kidneys, pancreas, and peritoneal cavity

Sturge-Weber syndrome

Pathophysiologic Abnormality

Capillary hemangiomas over trigeminal nerve distribution on face; may be linked with certain kinds of brain damage

Symptoms

Seizures if lesion involves optic branch of trigeminal nerve distribution

Physical Findings

Port-wine-stain due to capillary hemangiomas on face, glaucoma

Prognosis

Seizures may be intractable without surgical removal of part of the brain

Ataxia-Telangiectasia

Alternate Terminology

Louis-Bar syndrome

Etiology

Autosomal recessive inheritance

Pathophysiologic Abnormality

Affects skin, cerebellum and immune system

Symptoms

Ataxia usually in first 5 years of life

Physical Findings

Telangiectasias most prominent in second 5 years of life, and involve conjunctivae and ears

Potential Complications

Lung infections due to immunoglobulin A deficiency by age 10 years
Malignant lymphomas by age 15-20 years

Differential Diagnosis

Cerebral palsy, Friedreich's ataxia

Prognosis

Death usually occurs due to infection or malignancy

Degenerative Brain Diseases

Most diseases of this category are genetically transmitted and may involve metabolic derangements. While they are characterized by a deterioration of function, this deterioration may initially be manifest as arrested neurologic development.

Entities detectable by urine "metabolic screen" include:

Disease	Detected By
phenylketonuria (PKU)	Ferric chloride
maple syrup urine disease	Ferric chloride
hypothyroidism	TSH, T4
tyrosinosis	Ferric chloride
galactosemia	Benedict's solution
fructosemia	Benedict's solution
homocystinuria	Nitroprusside
hypermethionemia	Nitroprusside
mucopolysaccharidosis	Cetrimonium bromide

Degenerative diseases of the basal ganglia - reflected primarily via movement disorders such as dystonia, chorea, athosis, tremor:

Wilson's Disease
    Alternate Terminology
        Hepatolenticular degeneration
    Etiology
        Autosomal recessive disorder
    Pathophysiologic Abnormality
        Defect in copper metabolism causing copper accumulation in tissue, including the brain, liver and cornea
    Physical Findings
        Hepatomegaly, choreoathetoid movements, Kayser-Fleischer ring in cornea
    Laboratory Findings
        Copper level greater than 250 mcg/g of liver is diagnostic, decreased serum copper, decreased serum ceruloplasmin
    Potential Complications
        Progressive neurologic deterioration if untreated
    Therapeutic Plan
        Life-long therapy with D-penicillamine, a chelating agent

Others

Disease	Salient Features
Tourette syndrome	involuntary motor tics, onset between 5-10 years, obscene utterances may be present

Disease	Salient Features
Dystonia musculorum deformans	muscle spasms causing slow twisting movements - cause unknown
Lesch-Nyhan syndrome	self-mutilation, elevated uric acid due to purine metabolism defect, mental retardation, choreoathetosis

Degenerative decreases of the cerebellum, brain stem and spinal cord - usually reflected in an ataxic gait:

Disease	Salient Features
Friedreich's Ataxia	progressive ataxia, weakness and wasting of distal muscles, death usually due to cardiomyopathy by 30 years of age
Ramsay Hunt syndrome	dentate cerebellar ataxia
Hereditary cerebellar ataxias	familial occurrence

Degenerative diseases of the cerebral cortex white matter - manifest primarily by visual impairment and spasticity; dementia and seizures may occur late:

Disease	Salient Features
Metachromatic leukodystrophy	due to deficiency of the arylsulfatase A enzymes, infantile form fatal by age 5-6 years
Adrenoleukodystrophy	onset 8-10 years of age, death 2-5 years later, adrenal insufficiency with dementia and spastic gait
Rhett syndrome	occurs in girls, peculiar wringing motion of hands, progressive ataxia and dementia

Degenerative diseases of gray matter - many of this category are neuronal storage diseases:

Disease	Salient Features
Tay-Sachs disease	a gangliosidosis due to deficiency of hexosaminidase A, cherry red macula, hyperacusis to noise, death by 3-4 years of age
Niemann-Pick disease	due to accumulation of sphingomyelin in the reticuloendothelial system due to deficiency of sphinomyelinase, enlarged liver and spleen
Gaucher's disease	deficiency of glucocerebrosidase, hepatosplenomegaly
Menkes kinky hair disease	X-linked defect in copper absorption, death before 2 years of age, profound neurologic deficits

Neuromuscular Disorders

Anterior horn cell diseases:

Disease	Salient Features
Spinal muscular atrophy	similar to amyotrophic lateral sclerosis in adults
Werdnig-Hoffman disease	progressive disease, often fatal by 2 years

Diseases of the Neuromuscular Junction

Myasthenia Gravis
    Etiology
        Autoimmune disease with antibodies developing against acetylcholine receptors at the motor end-plate

Pathophysiologic Abnormality

Neonatal mysasthenia gravis - transient; due to transplacental antibodies from mother; resolves within 2 months

Congenital myasthenia gravis - antibodies are not detectable in this form; ptosis noted by 2 years of life

Juvenile myasthenia gravis - similar to adult form

Physical Findings

Muscle weakness which returns to normal with a edrophonium test

Chronologic Sequence of Events

If ocular muscle weakness alone is involved for more than 2 years, progression of the disease is limited

Therapeutic Plan

Pyridostigmine; immunosuppression with steroids may help

Peripheral Neuropathies

Guillain-Barré syndrome

Etiology

Typically follows viral infection or immunization

Pathophysiologic Abnormality

Demyelinizing polyneuropathy

Symptoms

Paresthesias may accompany the weakness

Physical Findings

Ascending muscle weakness/paralysis

Laboratory Findings

Elevated CSF protein with normal CSF cell count

Chronologic Sequence of Events

Recovery may take up to a year

Potential Complications

Respiratory failure, hypertension

Therapeutic Plan

Supportive care

Prognosis

Fatalities rare; 10-15% may have residual muscle deficits

Hereditary Sensory and Motor Neuropathy
    Alternate Terminology
        Charcot-Marie-Tooth disease (peroneal muscle weakness) is most common of this group
    Symptoms
        Weakness begins in feet in first decade of life
    Physical Findings
        Ataxia, retinitis, deafness
    Laboratory Findings
        Delayed nerve conduction time on EMG
    Prognosis
        May progress to significant loss of muscle strength, but most often is mild course with normal life expectancy

Morié Spencer

Developmental Considerations

Many skeletal deformities in infancy are due to positional pressures and force in utero and will resolve spontaneously.

After a breech or cephalic delivery, the hips will lie in flexion of 30-60 degrees. Also, there is knee contracture of 20 to 40 degrees and 10 to 30 degrees of internal tibial torsion.

Intrauterine postural deformities that can be manipulated back to normal position will generally spontaneously resolve by 3 months (in over 90% of infants).

Varum refers to angulation of a bone toward the midline. Genu Varum means "bowlegs", since the leg distal to the knee bends toward the midline. Valgum refers to angulation of the bone distal to a joint away from the midline. Genu Valgum means "knock-knee", since the bone distal to the knee angles away from the midline. From birth to about 18 months there is a normal stage of development in which "bowlegs" persists. After 24 months, children develop increasing valgus until, in adolescence, they finally have knees which are straight or with a minor degree of varus or valgus. Follow up and reassurance to parents are generally the only needed treatment for "bowlegs" or "knock-knees". Early walking is associated with valgus. Either entity may have a positive family history.

Developmental femoral anteversion (hip intoeing) presents between 2 and 6 years and is the most common cause of intoeing. Treatment usually is not needed and this will resolve with age. Internal tibial torsion is the second most common cause of intoeing. It is present between 3 months and 2 years. It is a result of intrauterine positioning and is common in normal children, especially neonates. No treatment is required.

Flat feet or flexible pronated feet commonly present at ages 3 to 7 years almost always without complaints, other than cosmetic. For many years various forms of treatment have been used to correct this "problem", including surgery. Two things to remember: the foot is not mature until around 12 years of age and no treatment (except surgery) has any permanent effect, and research suggests that even in severe cases, the flexible pronated adult is not disabled by the condition.

CHAPTER 16

Clinical Presentations

Acquired Injuries to Joints and Bones

The physis or growth plate is the main difference between young and mature bone.

The physis lies between the epiphysis and the metaphysis.

Because fractures that involve growth can have long-lasting consequences, there is a separate classification for immature bone.

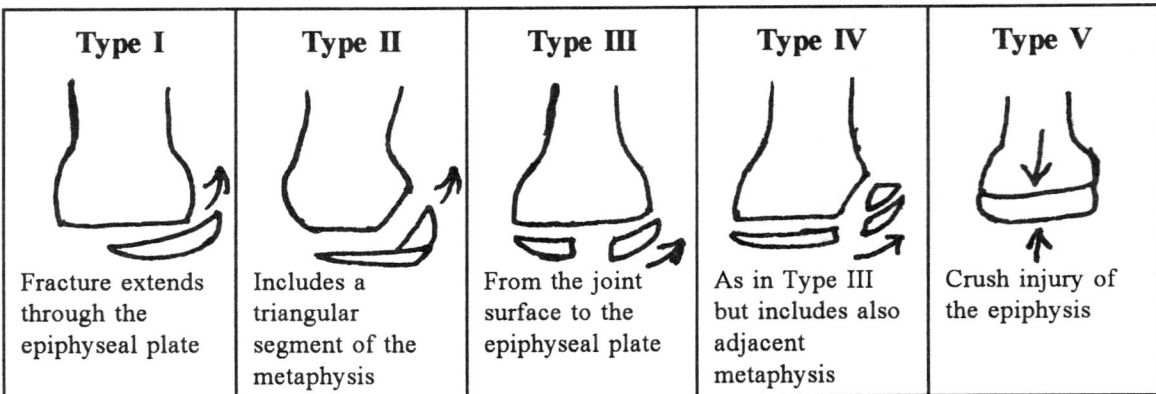

Type I	Type II	Type III	Type IV	Type V
Fracture extends through the epiphyseal plate	Includes a triangular segment of the metaphysis	From the joint surface to the epiphyseal plate	As in Type III but includes also adjacent metaphysis	Crush injury of the epiphysis

On X-rays, the bones of children can be "aged" based on the calcification of the epiphyses, which occurs on a bell curve distribution; so bone age as opposed to chronological age can be found. The two should correlate in most children. This is a useful tool in children with growth delay, etc.

Trauma

Fractures in children heal well; a careful exam to assure that no neurological or vascular injury has occurred is needed.

Neurologic - loss of or altered sensation; loss of function.

Vascular changes - decreased blood flow, cool pale extremity.

Both are emergencies and will likely need orthopedic consultation.

Fractures in children less than 2 years without a reasonable consistent story and any fracture in a child less than 1 year is suspicious for abuse.

Ankle injuries - generally, if they could support weight within 30 minutes of injury, even if they cannot now, it is a sprain not a fracture. Sprains are more common as the child's age increases.

Clavicle fractures are common and heal without problems; splint for comfort.

Generally, fractures that do not have neurovascular injuries and are not open can be splinted and definitively treated with casting in a few days when the swelling subsides. Exceptions are few that need surgical pinning to stabilize. Consult ortho if this occurs.

Sprain/Strain/Contusion - all involve some degree of tissue inflammation. Can be splinted for comfort, ice for the first 48 hours and NSAIDs.

Ligaments around joints are stronger than epiphyseal plates in children. Be wary of diagnosing sprains in joints that still have growth plates. Usually the epiphysis gives before the ligament.

Puncture wounds of the soles of the feet (especially through dirty tennis shoes) are prone to osteomyelitis (organism commonly *Pseudomonas aeruginosa*).

Lacerations of the feet often need splinting to maintain sutures in active children.

Infection

The child that refuses to bear weight (after exam and interview have lowered suspicion for fracture) must be considered as a possible septic joint.

Painless limps may present as changes in muscle tone, strength, or joint function. These may be caused by neurologic disease, muscle disease, bone and joint disorders, or hysteria.

Painful limps may be caused by trauma or infection (either of legs, or intra-abdominal processes (appendicitis)).

Lab is dictated by findings; children may be afebrile with osteomyelitis, especially of the feet.

Sedimentation rate is a sensitive, but not very specific test. However, if it is normal it moves osteo and septic joint down on the differential diagnosis.

Transient synovitis is common and presents as acute onset of a painful limp. It is typical between 4-10 years old; the child suddenly refuses to walk and may have a slightly elevated temperature. The sedimentation rate may be only slightly elevated. X-ray may be normal or show widening of the joint space. Often there is a history of viral illness in the recent past. Boys are affected 2:1. Because septic arthritis has to be considered, a joint aspiration must be done; lab studies in toxic synovitis are normal; it is a diagnosis of exclusion. Conservative treatment of bed rest is needed and the prognosis is very good.

Septic arthritis can be a devastating disease if not recognized and treated. It can occur in all ages from the newborn period onward. Clinically it presents as a painful joint with refusal to move the joint at all. Systemic symptoms are common. Sed. rate and WBC will normally be elevated, but direct needle aspiration of the joint is the most valuable test. Treatment is often surgical drainage with antibiotic therapy. Delayed treatment can result in joint destruction.

Osteomyelitis or infection of the bone occurs most frequently in younger children but can be seen at any age. Boys are affected 3:1. Spread is most commonly hematogenous, but can be by direct extension from soft tissue or direct external introduction (puncture wound). In children less than 18 months, where the physis has not yet formed, the infection can reach across the nonexistent growth plate to the epiphysis leading to septic arthritis. Pain is the most common symptom; patients may also have fever, localized erythema, and swelling. X-ray findings lag by 7-10 days; early findings are periosteal new bone formation. However, radionuclide bone scanning may be positive as early as 24-48 hours after abscess formation. Treatment, especially if diagnosed early, may be antibiotics. Surgical debridement and drainage may be necessary.

Common organisms in both septic arthritis and osteomyelitis:

Neonatal - Group B streptococcus, gram-negative enteric bacilli, also *Staphylococcus aureus*.

Toddlers and children - *Staphylococcus aureus*, streptococci, and *Haemophilus influenzae*.

Adolescence - same as children plus *Neisseria gonorrhoeae*.

With sickle cell disease - *Strep. pneumoniae* common, also salmonella.

Arthritis and Joint Pain in Children

Rheumatoid arthritis can occur at any age in childhood but the greatest prevalence is from 5 to 8 years old. It is an autoimmune disease which produces a rheumatoid factor, causing the release of lysosomal enzymes which breakdown the articular surface of a joint.

Three Forms:

Stills disease - a systemic multisystem disease with generalized arthritis, it is the most severe and is more frequent in young children.

Polyarticular arthritis - Common between 8-10 years with few systemic affects, this frequently involves fingers, spine, ankles, and feet.

Pauciarticular arthritis - seen through adolescence, the lower extremities are more often affected; about one half of cases are monarticular. Female more common with 2:1 ratio, this disease is worse in the morning; iridocyclitis occurs in 18% of cases. In absence of iridocyclitis, it is mostly benign.

Treatment for all three is NSAIDs and physical therapy.

Hemophiliacs may have hemarthrosis or bleeding into the joint causing synovial inflammation which with reoccurrence can lead to osteoarthritis. This generally occurs in a weight-bearing joint. Treatment is early diagnosis and IV transfusion of missing factor.

Sickle cell disease may first present as dactylitis in infants. There are radiographic changes secondary to the red marrow expansion. Also bony infarcts lead to increased bony trabeculation and sclerosis. The infarcted areas have a high risk of infection.

Neoplastic disorders can also present as bone or joint pain. Leukemia with neoplastic growth within the bone marrow may first present as bone pain. Ewing's sarcoma is most often in long bones; it is highly malignant.

CHAPTER 16

Common Regional Musculoskeletal Problems

General Musculoskeletal Disorders
Rickets
Rickets occurs when growing bone is inadequately mineralized and softens. Abnormality - the excessive osteoid formation causes widening of the metaphyses which results in the characteristic delay in linear growth, widening of wrists and knees, bowing of the legs and prominent costochondral junctions (rachitic rosary). Inadequate dietary vitamin D, lack of absorption of vitamin D due to fat malabsorption, of defects in vitamin D in the liver or kidney can all cause rickets.

Congenital Amputations
May be due to amniotic bands, teratogens, or rarely hereditary defects. Most are spontaneous and are not expected to recur in offspring.

Achondroplasia (Classic Chrondrodystrophy)
Heritable, the limbs are short, with the humerus and femur proportionately shorter than the radius and tibia. Varum deformities are usual. Moderate hydrocephalus, lumbar lordosis, short, stubby digits, restriction of motion of major joints are common. Mentality and sexual functions are normal.

Osteopetrosis (Albers-Schonberg Disease; Marble Bone Disease)
Heritable, the findings appear at any age. Characterized by pathologic fractures, myelophthisic anemia, splenomegaly, dwarfing, pigeon breast, square head, facial paralysis, auditory and visual disturbances. Calcification of soft tissues may occur.

Osteochondrodystrophy (Morquio's Disease)
A result of abnormal deposition of mucopolysaccharides, it is characterized by shortening of the spine, scoliosis, kyphosis, pigeon breast, hepatosplenomegaly, and corneal clouding. The child appears normal at birth and develops the deformities between 1 and 4 years of age. The condition is an autosomal recessive when familial.

Chondroectodermal Dysplasia (Ellis-Van Creveld Syndrome)
The condition is familial, and occurs more frequently in the Amish people of Pennsylvania. Mental retardation, ectodermal dysplasia, poor dentition, congenital heart disease, polydactyly, and syndactyly are major components of this syndrome.

Marfan's Syndrome
Characterized by unusually long digits (arachnodactyly) and hypermobility of the joints. High-arched palate, scoliosis, upward subluxation of ocular lenses, and iridodonesis are common. They have a high risk for thoracic aneurysms.

Arthrogryposis Multiplex Congenita

Involves fibrous ankylosis of most of the joints of the body with poor muscular development. Usually have normal mentaltion, but activity can be severely restricted.

Osteogenesis Imperfecta

Inheritance is usually autosomal dominant. Abnormality - In the severe fetal type (osteogenous imperfecta congenita) fractures may occur even in utero, and are common during birth. Growth retardation occurs because of recurrent fractures. Mentation is normal. Blue sclera are the characteristic finding.

Foot Problems

Posturing is the habitual position in which one holds the foot; however, it can be manipulated into normal position. A deformity is present if the foot cannot be manually manipulated into normal position.

Flatfoot (pes planus)

If a longitudinal arch is present when the child is not weight bearing, the arch will develop normally and no treatment is needed.

Cavovarus Foot

An unusually high longitudinal arch of the foot. Neurologic abnormalities such as Charcot-Marie-Tooth disease, Friedreich's ataxia, and diastematomyelia should be ruled out.

Pigeon Toes

Toeing in on the foot may be due to posturing or deformity of the foot, tibia, or femur.

Metatarsus Adductus

Positional deviation of the forefoot that can be corrected by manipulation. Serial castings may be needed to prevent development of a high arch with medial inclination of the heel.

Metatarsus Varus

Medical deformity of the forefoot that cannot be corrected by manipulation, due to an intrauterine subluxation of tarsometatarsal joints with adduction and inversion of the metatarsal bones. Serial casting or surgery may be needed to prevent development of a high arch with medial inclination of the heel.

Talipes Equinovarus (clubfoot)

The foot is pointed downward (like a horse: equinus=horse), with medial deviation of the forefoot and medial inversion of the heel. Spontaneous correction does not occur. Aggressive treatment is indicated. Those not responding to serial casting will require surgical correction.

Talipes Calceneovalgus

This is a benign condition due to intrauterine molding pressures. The foot is averted and dorsiflexed at the ankle. Passive stretching usually results in correction. The reverse of clubfoot.

Lower Leg Problems

Tibial Torsion

The tibia is normally internally rotated and bowed until about 9 years of age.

Blount's Disease

A disturbance of the growth plate at the proximal tibia. More common in those with precocious walking and African ancestry. If not corrected with braces and/or surgery, it can leave permanent deformities. May follow fractures involving the growth plates.

Osgood-Schlatter's Disease

Tenderness and swelling over the tibial tuberosity due to fibrocartilage microfractures at the insertion of the patellar tendon. It occurs in late childhood and early adolescence, and is more common in males. The condition is generally benign, but pain may persist with activity for up to a year after skeletal maturity.

Knee Problems

Osteochondritis Dessicans

This is the result of necrosis and separation of bone adjacent to articular cartilage. The knee is a common site for it to occur, though it can also be found in talus, femoral head, or lateral humeral condyle. The area is at risk for fractures.

Thigh Problems

Leg Length Discrepancies

Shortening of a femur is a common cause of discrepancies in leg length. Orthopedic evaluation is indicated if the difference in leg lengths is greater than 2.5 cm.

Hip Problems

Congenital Dysplasia of the Hip

In the newborn period the Barlow test (a click is felt as the hip is adducted toward midline in a flexed position) is diagnostic. The Ortolani test (the hip is abducted away from midline, producing a click if the femoral head slips out of the acetabulum) is the opposite of the Barlow test and is confirmatory. Asymmetric gluteal folds and apparent shortening of the affected leg are also clues to the presence of this condition. More common in girls. Whether the hip is dislocatable or dislocated, it needs to be detected and treated before the child walks or permanent deformity will ensue.

Slipped Capital Femoral Epiphysis

A fracture through the physis of the femoral head can occur during the pubescent growth spurt. Shortening of the thigh and loss of internal rotation of the hip are characteristic findings of this condition. The vulnerable age group: males 10-17 years; females 8-15 years. This condition is associated with the black race, males, obesity, and hypothyroidism.

Legg-Calve-Perthes Disease

Avascular necrosis of the femoral head. Persistent pain is common. The highest incidence is between 4 and 8 years of age, during the period of rapid growth of the epiphysis. The incidence is 6 times greater in males than females.

Toxic Synovitis

Transient synovitis is the most common cause of limps in boys in the 3 to 10 years age range. It often follows an URI and has a normal erythrocyte sedimentation rate and normal WBC. Because symptoms, age, sex, and laboratory are similar to that found in avascular necrosis of the hip and cannot always be distinguished from septic arthritis, serial hip X-rays or technetium bone scans and possibly joint aspiration are warranted.

Spine Problems

Scoliosis

Adolescent idiopathic scoliosis has its onset after 10 years of age and can progress rapidly during the pubescent growth spurt. Females are at high risk for progressive deformity. A history of pain should initiate search for lesions of the spinal cord or neoplasms, since the idiopathic condition is generally painless. Cases with curves more than 20 degrees should have orthopedic evaluation.

Torticollis

This condition is common in the neonatal period and is associated with a contracture of the sternocleidomastoid muscle. Torticollis may also be seen from gastroesophageal reflux (Sandifer syndrome) and with subluxation of cervical spine facettes. Hint: muscle spasm occurs on the side of shortening of the sternocleidomastoid in spastic torticollis and the opposite side in subluxation.

Klippel-Feil Anomaly

The result of segmentation failure in the cervical spine, this has a high association with other abnormalities, including cardiac lesions, urinary tract problems and auditory apparatus anomalies.

Diastematomyelia

The spinal cord is split and anchored in the spinal canal by bony or fibrous spicules. The result can be dysfunction of the bladder or lower extremity muscles. A hairy patch is often present over the affected area of the spine. A tethered spinal cord can produce similar problems.

Down Syndrome Subluxation of C1

Ligamentous laxity can occur in children with Down syndrome and place them at risk for subluxation of C1 or C2.

Elbow Problems

Subluxation of the Radial Head

Referred to as nursemaid's elbow, this condition can occur when the toddler is picked up by the wrist. The child typically holds the arm by his side with the palm down (pronated) and refuses to use it until it is reduced by supination of the palm while flexing the elbow.

Elbow Fracture

Suprachondylar fractures of the elbow are at high risk for development of compartment syndrome (Volkmann's contracture) if not adequately treated. Needs orthopedic consult.

Thomas A Lera
Jane E Puls

Management of a critically ill or injured child demands a systematic approach. This systematic approach must include a plan to identify and begin emergent treatment for stabilization of the patient even before a complete history and physical examination are obtainable. In addition, a timely, directed evaluation of each body area must be performed in order to minimize the chance of overlooking potentially serious additional/contributing illnesses or injuries.

The above is accomplished utilizing a PRIMARY and SECONDARY SURVEY system. The PRIMARY SURVEY is an initial assessment of the status of the patient's airway, oxygenation, ventilation, circulation and neurologic status. During this phase, life-threatening problems are identified and, because it is not uncommon to encounter serious physiologic alterations in the course of the primary survey, it is frequently necessary to interrupt the order of the survey to perform resuscitative measures. In contrast, the SECONDARY SURVEY includes a detailed, timely complete physical exam. It surveys each body area in a head-to-toe fashion. Included here are a directed history, a brief past medical history, indicated lab and/or radiographic studies which may lead to a specific diagnosis or a list of problems which may require further attention.

Mneumonics based on the ABCs can help guide one in the performance of both of these surveys.

Primary Survey

Airway

The goals of airway management are:
- Recognition and relief of obstruction
- Promotion of adequate gas exchange
- Prevention of aspiration of gastric contents
- Attention to protection of the cervical spine

Treatment/Therapeutic modalities:
- Triple Airway Maneuver: tilt head back, displace mandible forward open mouth (jaw thrust alone with suspected neck injuries - NOTE: the tongue is the most common obstruction to the pediatric airway)
- Use oral suction cautiously; may need oropharyngeal airway
- Endotracheal intubation; cricothyroidotomy

CHAPTER 17

Breathing/Ventilation

Observe for adequate gas exchange - look, listen, feel. Deficient air exchange must be rapidly diagnosed and treated. The following mneumonic addresses treatable causes of inadequate breathing:

Cause	Intervention
A irway obstruction	jaw thrust
T ension pneumothorax	aspiration/chest tube
O pen pneumothorax	aspiration/chest tube
M assive pneumothorax	aspiration/chest tube
F lail chest	positive pressure ventilation
C ardiac tamponade	pericardiocentesis
G astric distension	NG tube

Methods to Augment Ventilation
- Mouth to mask (over patients mouth/nose) breathing
- Bag-valve-mask ventilation
- Endotracheal intubation with mechanical ventilation
- Cricothyrotomy (needle/surgical)

Generous use of O_2 (100%) is warranted initially in almost all emergency settings. NOTE: Children will electively place themselves in a position of maximal airway comfort when allowed/able to do so. Do not change this position unnecessarily until more definitive airway/breathing measures are available.

Oxygen should be supplied by a means that meets the patient's needs, ie, percent of O_2 needed AND that is acceptable to the patient, eg: hood, nasal prongs, face mask, shield, cannula, etc.

Circulation

Assess overall circulatory status - note the quality, rate and regularity of the pulses - centrally and peripherally. Determine capillary refill time and blood pressure NOTE: blood pressure is an insensitive measure of adequate circulation in children until profound deficiencies exist - compromised circulation can and does exist despite a normal blood pressure.

Provide circulatory support; diagnose and control both external and internal hemorrhage:
- Control active hemorrhage - direct pressure
- IVF, crystalloid/colloid/blood
- MAST suit application (rarely truly appropriate in pediatrics)
- External cardiac massage (CPR)
- Defibrillation

Obtain reliable venous access: IV/IO access
> Blood for lab studies, including Type and Crossmatch

Disability (De-Brain)

Rapid screening of neurological system is essential. Obtain "neuro vital signs": assessment of pupillary response; level of consciousness [Alert, Verbal response, Pain response, Unresponsive]; notation of localized signs.

Calculation of Glasgow Coma Scale can be used.

Exposure/Environment

Complete physical exam requires the removal of all clothing. Children cool rapidly because of their large surface-to-body ratio. Maintain temperature by radiant warmer or warming blanket at 36-37° C.

Address hypo-hyperthermia as needed.

Foley Catheter

Do not place if blood at urinary meatus or with suspected pelvic fracture

Gastric Decompression - Orogastric/Nasogastric Tubes

Do not place if suspected facial fractures present. **Always** confirm placement.

History

Obtain an **A M P L E** history
> **A** llergies
> **M** edication
> **P** ast medical illness
> **L** ast medication
> **E** vents surrounding illness/injury

Secondary Survey

Detailed Physical Exam

Head (HEENT)
- Maxillofacial trauma - palpate bony prominences; evidence for bloody or CSF discharge from nose, mouth, ears; nasal septal hematoma; check dentition; suspect basilar skull fracture with Battle's sign, raccoon eyes, hemotympanum
- Dehydration - sunken fontanelle and/or eyes
- Eyes - pupillary size and reaction, visual acuity, fundal exam
- Scalp - exam for lacerations/hematomas
- Fontanelle   - sunken: dehydration
                 - bulging: may indicate increased ICP, meningitis/sepsis

Neck
> Palpate for obvious signs of fracture/dislocation and midline position of trachea; examine for SQ emphysema, hematoma, localized pain; assess for JVD; **[NECK/C-SPINE FILMS]**

Chest
- Evaluate visually for adequacy of respiratory excursion, asymmetry of chest wall motion or presence of a flail segment
- Carefully palpate chest wall and auscultate lung fields and heart
- R/O pulmonary/myocardial contusion, aortic/tracheobronchial/esophageal disruptions; **[CHEST FILMS]**
- Examine/assess respiratory adequacy by: skin color, nasal flaring, use of accessary muscles, grunting, stridor, wheezing, positioning of child

Abdomen
- Initial exam: inspect for ease of abdominal wall movement with respiration, gentle palpation, auscultation of bowel sounds.
- Observe and palpate flanks
- Serial examinations are often needed to establish a definitive diagnosis
- Investigate pregnancy and its related problems with female patients

Pelvis
- Palpate bony prominences for tenderness, instability
- Exam perineum for laceration, hematoma, acute bleeding or discharge
- Check urethral meatus for blood
- Child/sexual abuse

Rectum
  Evaluate integrity of wall, prostatic injury, muscle tone, occult GI hemorrhage; child abuse

Extremities
- Exam for signs of abrasion, contusion, hematoma, soft tissue injuries
- Exam for bony instability and neurovascular function
- Exam for fractures/dislocations

Back
  Exam with neck/spinal immobilization as indicated **NOTE:** this is accomplished if no obvious spinal cord injury or paralysis is present.

Skin
- Exam for bruises/petechiae - color, size, "age" may be suggestive of trauma, coagulopathy, physical abuse
- Rash - hemorrhagic, stellate, or rapidly expanding may indicate life-threatening illnesses (eg: meningococcemia, septic shock, anaphylaxis, etc)
- Burns
- Bites

Neurologic
- In-depth neuro exam: motor, sensory, cranial nerve and level of consciousness determinations
- Exam tympanic membranes, nose for basilar skull fracture
- Fundi exam
- Presence of spinal cord trauma

Detailed History

As appropriate and available

Radiographic and Lab Studies

Based on physical finding in 1°/2° survey and history; may need serial exams and more sophisticated studies, eg: computed tomography

Monitoring

Continuous monitoring and frequent reevaluation are a must

List Findings

Documentation of initial assessments and resuscitation procedures; list additional areas needing consultation/investigate

Definitive Care

In-hospital care; determine need for operative intervention and/or intensive care admission

Diagnostic Modalities/Pathophysiologic Considerations

Dependent on the patient's presentation and history, some of the following may be useful.

Indications for Intubation of the Comatose Child
- Inability to maintain patent airway
- Glasgow Coma Scale < 8
- Absent cough reflex
- Absent gag reflex
- Hypoxemia with adequate supplemental oxygen
- Hypoventilation
- Impending brainstem herniation (hyperventilation Rx)

Basic CPR in Infants and Children
(for children > 8 years: AHA recommends CPR be
performed as one would in an adult)

Infant	**Older Child**
(< 1 year)	(1-8 years)

Airway
Determine unresponsiveness
Call for help
Position patient supine
Support head and neck
Head-tilt/chin lift or jaw thrust
No blind finger sweeps

Breathing
2 initial breaths

Then: **20** breaths/min	Then: **15** breaths/min

Circulation
Check **brachial**/femoral pulse	Check **carotid**/femoral pulse

Activate EMS System

Compression rate: **100/min**	Compression rate: **80-100/min**

Compression:ventilation ratio = 5:1
Reassessment:palpate pulse every 10 cycles

Endotracheal Intubation (M-S-M-A-I-D)
All equipment at bedside and functioning

Mask	Appropriate size with bag and O_2
Suction	Tonsillar tip and tracheal
Machine	Appropriate for patient's size and problem
Airway	Laryngoscope, blade & ET tubes
	Tube size = 16 + age in years/4
	Tape, Benzoin
	< 8 years old, use uncuffed tube
IV	Patent and secure
Drugs	For intubation and resuscitation

Always check and re-check breath sounds following intubation.

Guidelines for Initiating Mechanical Ventilation
- Ventilator type: volume or pressure controlled
  NOTE: generally the type of ventilator and kind of support depend upon patient characteristics, eg: age, weight, reason for need for support, pathophysiology of disease process, time/point in disease process
- Initial Ventilator Settings
  * No Pulmonary Disease
    ▷ Pressure Ventilator
      ◇ Peak Pressure 16 - 24
      ◇ PEEP 0 - 5
      ◇ Rate Age Dependent
      ◇ I:E Ratio 1:1-1:2 (Never > 1 sec)
      ◇ FiO_2 ≤ 0.30
    ▷ Volume Ventilator
      ◇ Tidal Volume 8 - 15ml/kg
      ◇ PEEP 0 - 5
      ◇ Rate Age Dependent
      ◇ Insp Time (%) 25 - 33
      ◇ FiO_2 ≤ 0.30
  * With Pulmonary Disease
    ▷ Begin with ventilator set at above settings except $FiO_2 = 1.0$

▷ Adjust based upon
   ◇ Physical examination
   ◇ Non-invasive monitors: oximetry/capnography
   ◇ Arterial blood gases (Capillary blood gases)

Classification of Severity of Shock in Children

	I	II	III	IV
Estimated blood volume deficit	10-15%	15-30%	30-40%	>40%
Pulse (bpm)	>100	>120	>150	>150
Resp	normal	increased	marked increase	tachypneic/ apneic
Capillary refill (sec)	<4	> 4	> 6 - 8	> 10
Blood pressure	normal	narrowed pulse pressure	hypotensive	severely hypotensive to absent
Mentation	normal	anxious	confused	unconscious
Orthostatic hypotension	+	++	+++	++++
Urine output (ml/kg)	1-3	0.5-1	<0.5	none

Common Causes of Coma in Infants and Children

Pneumonic: TIPS on the Vowels

A --   **Alcohol:** Not only the adolescent patient is at risk for depressed levels of consciousness from alcohol. Infants may absorb enough alcohol through the skin from alcohol baths or from alcohol-containing medications to cause coma.

E --   **Epilepsy (and other causes of seizures):** Both postictal states and continued subtle seizure activity without overt motor manifestations can cause the appearance of coma in the infant and child.

I --   **Insulin (hypo- or hyperglycemia):** Infants without adequate hepatic glycogen stores or depressed gluconeogenesis may sucumb to hypoglycemia as the result of various disease processes. Hyperglycemia can also cause coma. A fingerstick glucose is indicated in all comatose children.

I --   **Intussusception:** A vacant blank stare is often seen in the child with intussusception.

O --   **Overdose:** Drug overdose may be intentional, accidental or the result of misguided attempts at recreational use. They can even be acquired transplacentally at birth. A toxic drug screen is indicated in all cases of coma without clear etiology.

U --   **Uremia (and other metabolic causes):** A serum ammonia and electrolytes are often helpful in providing clues to metabolic causes of coma.

T --   **Trauma:** In comatose infants, retinal hemorrhages should alert the examiner to the possibility of intracranial trauma due to a "shaken baby" or other form of abuse. Intracranial bleeds or cerebral edema resulting from trauma that caused hypoxia or shock may be assessed by a CT of the head.

I --   **Infection:** Infection is more common as a cause of altered sensorium in children than adults. A high index of suspicion should lead to a lumbar puncture as soon as the probability of increased intracranial pressure is excluded.

P --   **Psychiatric:** Factitious altered sensorium is exceedingly rare in children. It should be diagnosed by positive supporting evidence, not by lack of any other explanation for the an altered level of consciousness.

S --   **Stroke, shock, and other cardiovascular causes:** An altered level of consciousness can be caused by shock resulting in inadequate brain perfusion or by local cerebrovasular accidents. Hypertensive encephalopathy can cause a stroke like picture.

Glasgow Coma Scale

Response	Adults & Children	Infants	Points
Eye Opening	no response	no response	1
	to pain	to pain	2
	to voice	to voice	3
	spontaneous	spontaneous	4
Verbal	no response	no response	1
	incomprehensible	moans to pain	2
	inappropriate words	cries to pain	3
	disoriented conversation	irritable	4
	oriented and appropriate	coos, babbles	5
Motor	no response	no response	1
	decerebrate posturing	decerebrate posturing	2
	decorticate posturing	decorticate posturing	3
	withdraws to pain	withdraws to pain	4
	localizes pain	withdraws to touch	5
	obeys commands	normal spontaneous movements	6
Total Score			3-15

Evaluation and Management of Selected Pediatric Emergencies

Acute Respiratory Failure
   Criteria
>   RR >90/min (<12 mos)
>   RR >70/min (≥12 mos)
> P_aO_2 <40 torr (in absence of cyanotic heart disease)
> PCO_2 >65 torr
>   Mechanical Ventilation
>   Tracheal Intubation
   Definition
>   Clinical condition marked by inadequate O_2 elimination and/or inadequate oxygenation of blood

Etiologic Classification

- Lung Failure: diseases affecting airways, alveoli, capillary membranes, pulmonary circulation
    - * Upper airway obstruction
    - * Bronchiolitis
    - * Asthma
    - * Pneumonia
    - * Bronchopulmonary dysplasia
    - * Adult Respiratory Distress Syndrome
- Respiratory Pump Failure: disease along the pathway from brain stem to respiratory center to spinal cord, phrenic nerves to chest wall muscles
    - * Drug overdose
    - * CNS disease
    - * Neuromuscular disorders

Evaluation

- Physical exam is the most important tool
- Pulse oximetry (continuous/intermittent) gives information regarding oxygen saturation (O_2 sat <90 = PO_2 <60)
- Lab tests may include arterial blood gases, CXR

Signs & Symptoms

- Tachypnea/Dyspnea
- Intercostal Retractions
- Diminished Breath Sounds
- Cyanosis
- Altered sensorium

Blood Gas

- PO_2 <60 mm Hg (FIO_2 0.6)
- PCO_2 >45 mm Hg
- pH <7.3

Likely Underlying Causes

- Asthma (Hyperreactive Airways Disease)
- BPD (Bronchopulmonary Dysplasia)
- Bronchiolitis especially Respiratory Syncytial Virus
- ARDS (Adult Respiratory Distress Syndrome)
- Upper Airway Obstruction: CNS dysfunction; anatomic causes; infectious (croup, epiglottis); trauma; foreign body aspiration; burns; anaphylaxis/laryngospasm

Management

Mechanical ventilation

Shock
Definition
Syndrome of acute homeostatic derangement of various etiologies involving multiple organ systems, which ultimately causes failure of cellular metabolism. **NOTE:** shock is **not necessarily** decreased intravascular volume.

Criteria
- MAP <40 mm Hg (<12 mos)
- MAP <50 mm Hg $\geq$12 mos
- HR <50 BPM <12 mos
- HR <40 BPM $\geq$12 mos
- Cardiac arrest
- Need for continued vasoactive drug infusion

Etiology - Classification
- Hypovolemia - usually secondary to fluid or blood loss
  * Vomiting/diarrhea
  * Hemorrhagic
- Cardiogenic - hypoperfusion caused by heart failure (either inadequate filling or ejection)
- Neurogenic - diminished or absent CNS activity and loss of vascular tone
- Septic - shock from overwhelming bacteremia &/or septicemia

Signs and Symptoms
- Vasoconstriction
- Acrocyanosis
- Poor peripheral pulses
- Altered consciousness
- Pallor
- Sweating
- Ileus
- Oliguria

Differential Diagnosis of the "Shocky" Infant
- Infections
  * Meningitis
  * Bacterial sepsis
  * Viral infection
  * Urinary tract infection
- Cardiac
  * Dysrhythmias
  * Supraventricular tachycardia
  * Atrioventricular block
  * Congenital heart disease

*   Pulmonary hypertension
*   Cardiomyopathies
*   Myocarditis
*   Infiltrative disease
* Metabolic
  *   Electrolyte disturbances
  *   Hypoglycemia/hyperglycemia
  *   Inborn errors of metabolism
* Gastrointestinal
  *   Intestinal obstruction or ischemia
  *   Gastroenteritis with dehydration
  *   Vomiting
* Miscellaneous
  *   Child abuse
  *   Anemia
  *   Hepatic failure
  *   Intracranial bleed

Treatment
* Hypovolemic - fluid resuscitation
* Cardiogenic - vasopressors
* Neurogenic - Trendelenberg position, fluids, vasopressors
* Septic - fluids, vasopressors, antibiotic/antiviral therapy

Congestive Heart Failure
    Definition
        Inability of heart to pump adequate blood volume for the circulatory and metabolic needs of the body
    Etiology
* Commonly it results from:
  * Volume overload - increased preload or excessive intravascular volume
  * Pressure overload - increased afterload or increased vascular resistance
  * Myocardial dysfunction - $2°$ congenital lesions or acquired cardiomyopathy or myocarditis
  * Dysrhythmias

- Ninety percent of children who develop congestive heart failure do so in the 1st year of life as a result of congenital heart disease.
- Other etiologies include:
  * Cor pulmonale from chronic lung disease (eg: bronchopulmonary dysplasia)
  * Cardiomyopathy
  * Electrolyte abnormalities
  * Endocarditis or rheumatic carditis
  * Renal failure
  * Systemic hypertension
  * Anemia
  * Hyperthyroidism
  * Overhydration

Signs and Symptoms
- Decreased exercise tolerance
- Altered behavior
- Weight loss
- Change in eating habits
- Tachycardia
- +/- gallop rhythm
- Cardiomegaly
- Venous congestion (hepatomegaly, JVD, edema)
- Tachypnea with crackles
- Rhonchi
- Wheezing
- Orthopnea
- Exercise intolerance

Diagnosis
- Chest X-ray
- Electrocardiography
- Arterial blood gas
- Echocardiography

Management - Improve contractility while reducing afterload.
- Inotropic Agents
  * Digitalis
  * Fluids
  * Dopamine/Dobutamine
- Reduction of Preload (Volume Overload)
  * Fluid restriction
  * Diuretic therapy

- Reduction of Afterload (Pressure Overload)
  * Sodium nitroprusside

Altered Mental Status
Classification/Definitions
- Stupor: state of unresponsiveness - patient can be aroused by vigorous stimulation
- Coma: state of unresponsiveness - patient **cannot** be aroused Unresponsive)

  NOTE: Altered levels of consciousness, stupor and coma are signs of "brain failure" and should be treated emergently in an effort to minimize irreversible CNS injury.

Criteria for CNS Failure
- Glasgow Coma Scale < 5
- Fixed, Dilated pupils
- ICP > 20 torr (for > 20 min)

Managment Goals
- Prevent secondary hypoxic-ischemic brain injury
- Prevent herniation
- Diagnosis and treatment (if possible) of underlying cause of coma

Spinal Cord Trauma
Pediatric spinal cord injuries are unusual. They are most commonly seen with MVA (motor vehicle accidents) in < 10 year old age group; in those > 10 years - MVAs as well as recreational and organized sporting accidents account for the majority of spinal cord injuries

Evaluation
- History - A spinal injury should be assumed until proved otherwise in any comatose child. Children who are awake and complaining of neck or back pain or radicular pain, dysesthesias or numbness also are possible candidates for a spinal injury.
- Examination - Palpate for tenderness of the neck or spine in awake older children. A careful evaluation of the movement of the extremities, sensation, and reflexes in awake children should be done.
- Any child who is awake and flaccid has a spinal cord injury until proven otherwise.
- Hypotension can result from loss of vasomotor tone due to a cervical cord injury.

Management
* Immobilization
* Airway protection
* Blood pressure support
  NOTE: The early use of relatively high-dose steroids is advocated for some spinal cord injuries. Prompt neurosurgical intervention should be obtained when these patients are encountered.

Acute Renal Failure (AFR)
Criteria
BUN > 100 mg/dl
Serum Creatinine > 2 mg/dl
Dialysis
Diagnosis and Management
See Chapter 13 on Renal Disorders

Hypertensive Crisis
Hypertension in children is rare but should not be missed. It is defined as systolic, diastolic or mean arterial pressures that fall above the upper limit of normal (> 95%) for the patient's age. Careful attention must be given to the proper technique used to obtain blood pressure - especially in infants and small children.
Classification
* Hypertensive emergency
  * This condition has life-threatening end organ (CNS, cardiac, renal) involvement and needs to be corrected within minutes to hours.
  * Hypertensive encephalopathy
  * Malignant hypertension
  * Acute complications of accelerated hypertension
    ▷ Pulmonary edema
    ▷ Cerebrovascular accident with hemorrhage or infarction
  * Eclampsia
  * Pheochromocytoma
* Hypertensive urgency
  * No evidence of life-threatening end organ involvement; needs to be corrected in hours to days.
    ▷ Renal failure or impairment
    ▷ Acute glomerulonephritis
    ▷ Preeclampsia
    ▷ Postoperative bleeding
    ▷ Newly developed hypertension

Assessment

- Do not use too small a blood pressure cuff. The width of bladder on the blood pressure cuff should be at least 2/3 the length of the upper arm.
- Obtain a history to uncover possible underlying etiology of the hypertension (eg: renal disease, coarctation, pheochromocytoma, Cushing's disease, drug effect, neurofibromatosis).
- Physical exam should include four-extremity blood pressures, evaluation for end organ injury such as funduscopic changes, decreased visual acuity, congestive heart failure, abdominal bruit, motor or sensor disturbances, and potential causes such as cafe au lait spots.
- Obtain urinalysis, electrolytes BUN, creatinine, chest X-ray, EKG and if CNS involvement, a CT of the head. If the patients condition permits consider obtaining renin level prior to beginning antihypertensive therapy.
- Patients with blood pressure >95th percentile require further evaluation and may require therapy. Patients with evidence of target organ injury (eg: headache, vomiting, epistaxis, decreased visual acuity, funduscopic changes, congestive heart failure, proteinuria) or blood pressure significantly >95th percentile require immediate monitoring and treatment. NOTE: In patients being evaluated for **Hypertensive Cerebrovascular Syndromes**: when a patient presents with hypertension and an alteration in mental status - the hypertension work-up and emergent control should take precedent over the work-up for the change in mental status. Entities associated with HTCVS include: hypertensive encephalopathy, intracerebral hemorrhage, subarchnoid hemorrhage, head/neck trauma, side effects from recreational drugs and neoplasms.
- If possible, secure IV access before beginning therapy. (Nifedipine can be given sublingually to vomiting patients).

Etiology (Common Causes By Age)

- Neonate
  - * Coarctation of aorta
  - * Renovascular disease
  - * Intracranial hemorrhage
- Infants ≤ 2 yrs
  - * Renovascular disease
  - * Intrinsic renal disease
  - * Coarctation of aorta
  - * Neuroblastoma
- 2-8 yrs
  - * Renovascular disease
  - * Intrinsic renal diagnosis

- \> 8 yrs
  - * Renovascular disease
  - * Intrinsic renal disease
  - * Essential hypertension

Treatment

- Blood pressure should not be decreased by greater than one third of the total goal over the first 4-6 h.
- Patients with underlying chronic hypertension may have a shifted autoregulatory curve and require increased blood pressures to maintain normal cerebral perfusion. Therefore, elevated pressure should be lowered more slowly in these patients.
- Drugs

Drug	Dose	Comments
Diazoxide arteriolar vasodilator	1-3 mg/kg rapid IVP (undiluted) q 15-20 min x 2-3 doses	First line drug. May be given in ER setting NOTE: give with furosemide to avoid rebound hypertension.
Labetalol alpha and beta blocker	1-3 mg/kg/hr IV	First line drug. May require ICU setting
Nitroprusside arteriolar and venous vasodilator	0.5-8.0 mcg/kg/min IV	Very short half-life Allows tight control of BP reduction. Requires ICU monitoring.
Hydralazine arteriolar vasodilator	0.1-0.2 mg/kg IV	Second line drug. Maintains cerebral, renal, coronary, and uterine perfusion.
Phentolamine alpha blocker	0.1-0.2 mg/kg IV Increase dose as needed Effective dose may vary among patients	Use in suspected excess catecholamine states.
Nifedipine Ca^{++} channel blocker	0.25-0.5 mg/kg SL	Can be given SL in vomiting patients.
Minoxidil arteriolar vasodilator	2.5-5.0 mg PO	Consider in refractory renovascular hypertension

Hyperkalemia
Etiology
- Cell breakdown
- Renal failure
- Leukocytosis
- Transfusion with aged blood
- Hypoaldosteronism
- Thrombocytosis >750K/mm^3
- Aldosterone insensitivity
- Metabolic acidosis
- NaCl substitutes

- Cell lysis from blood drawing
- Decreased insulin
- K-sparing diuretics

Symptoms
- Apathy, weakness, paresthesias
- Tetany, carpalspasm
- ECG changes - T-wave elevation, loss of P-wave, widening of QRS, S-T depression, bradycardia, arrhythmia, cardiac arrest

Treatment

Drug	Dose and route	Onset (duration)	Mode of action	Comment
Calcium Gluconate 10% (100mg/ml)	20 mg/kg IV over 5 minutes may repeat x 2	Immediate (30-60 min)	Stabilizes Cell Membranes	CaCl can worsen acidosis Monitor for bradycardia Hold infusion if heart rate drops < 100.
Sodium Bicarbonate 7.5% (1mEq/cc)	1-2 mEq/kg IV	20 min (1-4 hours)	Enhances intracellular transport of K	Assure adequate ventilation Will precipate if given with Calcium.
Glucose + Insulin	1-2 g/kg (5-10cc/kg 20% dextrose) 0.3 units/g glucose Adminster by infusion together over 2 hours	15-30 min (3-6 hours)	Enhances intracellualar transport of K	Monitor blood glucose
Sodium polystyrene sulfonate (Kayexalate)	1 g/kg P.O. in 70% sorbitol or P.R. in 30% sorbitol every 6 hours		Exchanges K for Na in the intestine	Monitor for sodium overload
Dialysis		Time required for vascular access	Removes K from serum	Can also correct metabolic acidosis and fluid overload problems

Gastrointestinal Hemorrhage

Blood loss in excess of 20cc/kg in 24 hours, or the equivalent need in blood/fluid replacement, constitutes GI failure and demands prompt diagnosis and treatment interactions.

CHAPTER 17

Compartment Syndrome (CS)

This syndrome develops because of increased compartment contents in a limiting fascial envelope. Increased contents can be from hemorrhage and cellular swelling from ischemia or blunt trauma. When compartment pressure is greater than capillary perfusion pressure, ischemia further complicates/aggravates compartment swelling. Obvious sequalae included distal vascular and neuro problems.

Evaluation - Clinical signs of CS described as the "5 Ps":

- Pain is out of proportion to that expected. The most sensitive finding in the physical exam is exquisite pain with passive stretch of the involved muscles.
- Paresthesia arises from sensory nerves contained in the compartment.
- Pallor occurs in the distal part of the extremity due to poor capillary refill (> 3 seconds).
- Pulselessness in the distal extremity is a very late sign.
- Paralysis is also a late sign; early weakness should be sought instead.
  Note: CS is suspected even if only **one** of the above findings is present. Assessment relies on the accurate measurement of compartment pressure.

Treatment - Fasciotomy

Open Fractures

Management

- Cultures should be obtained from the wound as soon as possible on presentation in the emergency room.

- Antibiotic therapy: Include antistaphycoccal coverage (eg, a cephalosporin).

- For severely contaminated, massive crush - or farm injuries: Add gentamicin and penicillin for gram-negative rod and streptococcal coverage.
- Early operative debridement and irrigation is indicated in most cases, within 6 hours of injury.
- Tetanus prophylaxis

Jefry L Biehler
A Eugene Osburn

Developmental Considerations

Poisonings and drug overdoses are common problems encountered by physicians caring for children. It is estimated that approximately 1.5 to 3 million poisonings occur in the United States each year. Sixty percent of these poisonings occur in children under the age of 5.

The optimum management of the poisoned or overdosed patient requires an organized approach of evaluation and treatment. This management should always focus on the patient first and the poison second. The stabilization of vital signs, including the establishment and maintenance of the ABCs (airway, breathing, circulation) is the first priority in all poisoned patients. This should be followed by an attempt to identify the responsible toxin, specific therapy if warranted, decontamination if indicated, and appropriate ongoing treatment or observation.

Diagnostic Modalities

Patient History and Physical Examination

A majority of patients (including pediatric patients) will present for evaluation or treatment with the ingestion of a known toxic substance. For these patients the identification of the toxin and suggested management strategies may be found in numerous texts and widely available computer-based systems. For those patients presenting with an unknown ingestion or toxic exposure the history, physical examination, and proper laboratory tests frequently enable the physician to correctly identify the substance and provide necessary medical treatment.

If the patient is able to answer questions the physician should direct the history toward the identification of the ingested substance. An attempt to quantify the amount of toxic exposure, the elapsed time since exposure, and the development of symptoms since exposure should be elicited. For pediatric patients, available caretakers should be questioned. Questions should address the presence of household medications (prescription, over-the-counter and elicit drugs), other potential household toxins (cleaning compounds, plants, etc), and possible environmental exposures (insecticides, herbicides, fertilizers).

Toxidromes

A combination of findings from a careful history and physical examination may allow physicians to clinically classify toxic ingestions into one of the common autonomic syndromes. These autonomic syndromes, often referred to as "Toxidromes", may be used as a basis for empiric treatment of ingestions prior to laboratory identification of specific toxins.

The four most commonly recognized Toxidromes are listed below:

Sympathomimetic Syndrome

Physical examination findings and symptoms:

> Blood pressure elevated
> Heart rate elevated (except with severe hypertension)
> Pupils dilated
> Sweating
> Mental status changes (confused, anxious)
> Agitated
> Elevated temperature

Common substance ingestions associated with the sympathomimetic syndrome:

> Cocaine
> Amphetamines
> PCP
> Phenylpropanolamine

Sympatholytic Syndrome

Physical examination findings and symptoms:

> Blood pressure elevation
> Bradycardia
> Small pupils
> Mental status changes (obtunded, comatose)
> Decreased body temperature
> Decreased intestinal peristalsis

Common substance ingestions associated with the sympatholytic syndrome:

> Ethanol
> Barbiturates
> Sedative-hypnotics
> Clonidine
> Opioids

Cholinergic Syndrome

Physical examination findings and symptoms associated with the stimulation of Muscarinic receptors

S	Salivation (and Bronchorrhea)
L	Lacrimation
U	Urination
D	Diaphoresis
G	Gastrointestinal hyperperistalsis
E	Excitement (CNS) [from seizures to coma]
D	Decreased pupils, heart rate

Physical examination findings and symptoms associated with the stimulation of Nicotinic receptors:

> Initial hypertension and tachycardia
> Fasciculations and muscle weakness

Common substance ingestions associated with the cholinergic syndrome:

> Organophosphates
> Carbamates
> Physostigmine
> Nicotine

Anticholinergic Syndrome

Physical examination findings and symptoms:

Tachycardia
Hypertension
Elevated temperature
Dilated pupils
Flushed, hot, dry skin
Decreased intestinal peristalsis
Urinary retention
Myoclonic jerking
Choreoathetoid movements
Mental status changes (agitated delirium)

Common substance ingestions associated with the anticholinergic syndrome:

Antihistamines
Cyclic antidepressants
Atropine
Scopolamine
Phenothiazines

Odor Identification

Occasionally the identification of an ingested toxic substance is facilitated by the characteristic odor associated with the substance. The sensitivity of this method of toxin identification is very dependent on the observer. The following are some odors caused by toxins and drugs:

•	Acetone	Chloroform, Diabetic Ketoacidosis
•	Bitter almonds	Cyanide
•	Garlic	Arsenic, organophosphates
•	Mothballs	Naphthalene
•	Wintergreen	Methyl salicylate

Laboratory

Urine drug screening is often a useful tool in determining the presence of a specific ingested substance. However, many authorities argue that the routine use of these screens without regard to available clinical and historical patient information is on inefficient method of patient management. Toxidrome-oriented drug screening is a more cost and time-efficient utilization of toxicologic testing.

The **anion gap** is another laboratory measurement utilized in the evaluation of poisoned patients. The anion gap is calculated as follows:

$$\text{Anion Gap} = [\text{Na}] - ([\text{HCO}^3] + [\text{Cl}])$$

$$\text{Normal Anion Gap} = 8 - 12$$

The anion gap is a method of quantifying the presence of anions not measured by routine laboratory tests. A patient with metabolic acidosis may therefore be further described as having an elevated, normal, or reduced anion gap.

A simple way of remembering the common drugs or poisons causing an elevated anion gap is using the phrase AT MUD PILES.

A	Alcohols
T	Toluene
M	Methanol
U	Uremia
D	DKA (Diabetic Ketoacidosis)
P	Paraldehyde
I	Isoniazid, Iron, Ibuprofen
L	Lactic acid
E	Ethylene glycol
S	Salicylates

Another commonly measured "gap" in the evaluation of poisoned or overdosed patients is the **osmolar gap**. Serum osmolality may be measured in the laboratory by one of two methods. The first method utilizes the freezing point depression osmometer to determine osmolality. The second method uses a heat of vaporization method to determine osmolality. When measuring serum osmolality in the poisoned patient it is advisable to utilize the freezing point method. Alcohols may "boil off" before the serum osmolality is determined if the heat of vaporization method is used, thus giving a falsely normal osmolar gap.

$$\text{Calc. Osmolality} = 2[Na] + [glucose]/2 + [BUN]/2.8 = 285\text{-}295 \text{ mosm/L}$$

Osmolar gap = measured - calculated osmolality

A simple way of remembering the common drugs or poisons causing an elevated osmolar gap is using the phrase MEAN PIE.

M	Mannitol, Methanol
E	Ethanol, Ethyl ether
A	Acetone
N	"No Kidneys" (Renal failure without dialysis)
P	Propylene glycol
I	Isopropyl alcohol
E	Ethylene glycol

X-ray Identification

Abdominal X-rays may reveal radiopaque ingested substances. Recently ingested iron-containing tablets may be seen on plain X-rays. The sensitivity of this method for determining the presence of ingested materials is too low to make this a routine part of the evaluation of poisoned patients.

Therapeutic Considerations

Decontamination

The process of decontamination is usually divided into three areas: Decontamination of the
- Eyes
- Skin
- Gastrointestinal tract

Skin Decontamination

Because many toxins are rapidly absorbed through the skin (ie, organophosphates) the removal of these substances from the skin surface should be undertaken expeditiously. Contaminated clothing should be removed and the contaminated skin flushed with large amounts of water or saline. Care must be taken to avoid exposure of health care personnel during the decontamination process.

Eye Decontamination

Large volumes of warm water or saline should be used to flush the eyes of persons with toxic exposure of the eyes.

Gastrointestinal Decontamination

There is an ongoing controversy regarding the use of gastric decontamination in the poisoned patient. Many authors feel that the use of induced emesis or gastric lavage is only minimally effective in reducing the dosage of ingested substances. Many authors feel that the use of activated charcoal without prior gastric emptying is a more effective method of gastrointestinal decontamination. However the routine use of induced emesis and gastric lavage is still a common practice among physicians caring for overdosed patients.

Induced Emesis

The most common method of inducing emesis in the overdosed/poisoned patient is the administration of syrup of ipecac. This medication acts by both direct gastric mucosal irritation and by effects on the central nervous system. Although not recommended by most authors, apomorphine, an opiate derivative, is also effective in inducing emesis.

Contraindications for inducing emesis in poisoned patients are as follows:

- Patients in a coma or depressed neurologic condition
- Patients who have ingested substances which may result in sudden deterioration of mental status
- Patients with a depressed or absent gag reflex
- Patients who are having seizures
- Patients who have ingested caustics
- Patients who have ingested hydrocarbons

CHAPTER 18

Gastric Lavage

Gastric lavage with a large-bore nasogastric or orogastric tube is probably slightly more effective at removing ingested substances than induced emesis. The complications associated with this method of decontamination are listed below:

- Perforation of the esophagus or stomach
- Aspiration of stomach contents during placement
- Inadvertent tracheal intubation with the gastric tube
- Trauma to the nares or oral mucosa during placement
- Patient discomfort during tube placement

Activated Charcoal

The administration of activated charcoal as a liquid slurry is an effective method of intestinal decontamination. Activated charcoal is very absorbent of most common poisons and drugs. The large surface area produced in the activation process allows the charcoal to absorb significant amounts of ingested substances. Charcoal is indicated most all ingestions. Although some substances are poorly adsorbed by activated charcoal (iron, lithium, cyanide, alcohols, acids and bases) the potential advantage usually outweighs potential risks. The contraindications for the administration of charcoal are listed below:

- Patients who are to undergo endoscopy for manual removal of ingested substances.
- Patients with ileus or intestinal obstruction

Cathartics

Cathartics are used to hasten the elimination of poisons or ingested substances from the gastrointestinal tract. Substances used to decrease gastrointestinal transit time include the following:

- Magnesium citrate
- Sorbitol
- Polyethylene glycol solutions

The contraindications for cathartic administration are listed below:

- Patients with ileus or intestinal obstruction
- Comatose, convulsing or obtunded patients

Specific Indications for Hemodialysis	
Lithium	> 4.0 mEq/L
Salicylates	> 100 mg/dl
Methanol	> 50 mg/dl
Ethylene glycol	> 50 mg/dl

A number of specific antidotes are available for the treatment of selected toxins.

Toxin	Antidote
Acetaminophen	N-acetylcysteine
Atropine	Physostigmine
Arsenic	Dimercaprol
Benzodiazepines	Flumazenil
Carbon monoxide	Oxygen
Digoxin	Digitalis antibodies
Ethylene glycol	Ethanol
Heparin	Protamine
Iron	Deferoxamine mesylate
Lead	Dimercaprol, $CaNa_2$ - EDTA
Mercury	Dimercaprol
Methanol	Ethanol
Nitrates	Methylene Blue
Opiates	Naloxone
Organophosphates	Pralidoxime
Zinc	EDTA

Potentially Toxic Acute Doses of Selected Poisons

Toxin	Potentially Toxic Ingestion	Lethal Ingestion
Acetaminophen	150 mg/kg	
Iron	> 60 mg/kg	
Salicylates	100 mg/kg	
Ethylene glycol		1 - 1.5 ml/kg
Methanol		0.5 ml/kg

Disease Profiles

Acetaminophen Poisoning
   Etiology
      Acute ingestion of greater than 140 mg/kg of acetaminophen; chronic ingestion of greater than 150 mg/kg/day on 2 or more consecutive days.
   Pathophysiologic Abnormality

Stage	Time After Ingestion	Findings
I	1/2 - 24 hr	anorexia, nausea, vomiting, malaise, pallor, diaphoresis
II	24 - 48 hr	abdominal pain, liver tenderness, elevated liver enzymes, oliguria
III	72 - 96 hr	peak hepatic enzyme abnormalities, increased bilirubin, prolonged prothrombin time
IV	4 days-2 wks	resolution of hepatic toxicity or progressive hepatic failure

   Laboratory Findings
      Liver aminotransferase (AST or ALT) above 1,000 IU/L if hepatoxicity present. Note: Use the Rumack-Matthew nomogram to assess hepatotoxicity risk.
   Potential Complications
      Hepatic failure
   Diagnostic Plan
      Serum acetaminophen level: If elevated use serial determinations, liver enzymes.

Therapeutic Plan

Gastric decontamination within 4 hours of ingestion. Activated charcoal. N-acetylcysteine 140 mg/kg followed by 17 doses of 10 mg/kg every 4 hours.

Prognosis

Depends on progressing of hepatic toxicity.

Aspirin Poisoning

Alternate Terminology

Salicylism

Etiology

Acute ingestion: 150-300 mg/kg (mild symptoms); 300-500 mg/kg (moderate symptoms); > 500 mg/kg (severe symptoms or death)

Pathophysiologic Abnormality

Respiratory center stimulation (respiratory alkalosis); inhibition of Krebs cycle; uncoupling of oxidative phosphorylation; coagulopathies.

Predisposing Conditions

Due to inhibited platelet function and disturbances in vitamin K-dependent clotting factors; lactic and ketoacidosis (large anion gap metabolic acidosis) inhibition of glucose homeostasis.

Symptoms

Fever, nausea, vomiting, tachypnea, lethargy, slurred speech, seizures, tinnitus, diaphoresis.

Physical Findings

Kussmaul respirations, CNS depression, agitation, coma, seizures, cardiovascular collapse.

Laboratory Findings

Hyperglycemia, hypoglycemia, hypokalemia; coagulation abnormalities, metabolic acidosis with increased anion gap

Chronologic Sequence of Events

Tachypnea → respiratory alkalosis → metabolic acidosis → CNS depression → cardiovascular collapse.

Potential Complications

The respiratory alkalosis phase is relatively short in children; children usually present with metabolic acidosis.

Differential Diagnosis

Diabetic ketoacidosis, ethylene glycol ingestion, iron intoxication

Diagnostic Plan
　　Serum salicylate level, Chem 18, arterial blood gases, CBC
Therapeutic Plan
　　Supportive care, gastric decontamination; fluid resuscitation, alkalization of urine with sodium bicarbonate, potassium replacement, hemodialysis if salicylate level > 100 mg/dl.
Prognosis
　　Serum levels above 500 mg/dl often result in death in spite of treatment.

Methanol Poisoning
　Etiology
　　Antifreeze, windshield de-icers, solvent, stove fuels, paint removers
　Pathophysiologic Abnormality
　　Methanol is toxic when metabolized to formaldehyde and formic acid, which occurs over several hours (giving a latent period of 8-24 hours). Severe metabolic acidosis with anion and osmolar gaps occur. Amounts greater than 0.5 ml/kg can be fatal. Ethanol blocks methanol conversion to toxic substrates by binding to alcohol dehydrogenase sites.
　Symptoms
　　Headache, malaise, dizziness, parasthesia, blindness, CNS depression, abdominal pain.
　Physical Findings
　　Retinal hyperemia progressing to pale avascular retina, cardiac arrhythmias, seizures, reduced visual acuity.
　Laboratory Findings
　　Metabolic acidosis (CO_2 content may approach zero)
　　Methanol levels above 20 mg/dl are associated with toxicity
　　Methanol levels can be estimated by the formula osmolar gap x 3
　Chronologic Sequence of Events
　　Latent period of 8-24 hours
　Potential Complications
　　Blindness, death
　Differential Diagnosis
　　Other causes of metabolic acidosis with anion gap and osmolar gap.
　Diagnostic Plan
　　Chem 18, freezing point osmolality, methanol level, arterial blood gases
　Therapeutic Plan
　　Sodium bicarbonate, folic acid, ethanol to maintain a serum ethanol level at or above 100 mg/dl. Hemodialysis if serum methanol level > 50 mg/dl.

Prognosis

Permanent blindness correlates with severity of metabolic acidosis.

Ethylene Glycol Poisoning

Etiology

Antifreeze, radiator fluid, windshield de-icers

Pathophysiologic Abnormality

The parent state is non-toxic. Metabolism by alcohol dehydrogenase produces toxic intermediates, including glycoaldehyde, glycolic acid (causing metabolic acidosis) and calcium oxalate crystals (damaging all vital organs). Toxicity appears within hours of ingestion.

Symptoms/Physical Findings

Stage	Time After Ingestion	Findings	Mechanism
I		CNS changes, nausea, vomiting, coma, seizures, hypercalcemia, crystalluria, tetany, rhythm disturbances	Profound metabolic acidosis, formation of calcium oxalate
II		coma, cardiopulmonary failure	acidosis, hypocalcemia
III	24 - 72 hr	renal failure	acute tubular necrosis

Laboratory Findings

Hypocalcemia, severe metabolic acidosis, urine may fluoresce under Woods lamp (if due to radiator antifreeze), oxalate crystals in urine.

Differential Diagnosis

Diabetic ketoacidosis, other alcohols.

Diagnostic Plan

CBC, UA, Chem 18, serum osmolarity, ethylene glycol level

Therapeutic Plan

Sodium bicarbonate, calcium, pyridoxine and thiamine, ethanol to produce serum level at or above 100 mg/dl.

Prognosis

Depends on end-organ impairment.

Isopropryl Alcohol Poisoning

    Etiology

        Ingestion, dermal absorption

    Pathophysiologic Abnormality

        Metabolized to acetone. Does not cause metabolic acidosis, causes myocardial depression, hypotension and shock.

    Symptoms

        Intoxication, gastritis

    Physical Findings

        CNS depression

    Laboratory Findings

        Osmolar gap

    Potential Complications

        Cardiovascular collapse

    Differential Diagnosis

        Coma, ketonuria and absence of metabolic acidosis strongly suggest the diagnosis

    Diagnostic Plan

        Serum osmolarity, arterial blood gases, urinalysis

    Therapeutic Plan

        Supportive; hemodialysis if hemodynamically unstable

    Prognosis

        Death can occur at blood levels above 400-500 mg/dl

Ethanol Poisoning

    Etiology

        Most frequently ingested alcohol

    Pathophysiologic Abnormality

        In adolescents, levels of 100-150 mg/dl cause intoxication and mild neurologic symptoms; levels above 500 mg/dl may be lethal.

        In children, levels above 50-100 mg/dl cause coma, hypoglycemia and hypothermia. Blood alcohol levels of 100 mg/dl result from 10-15 ml/kg of beer (5% alcohol), 4-6 ml/kg of wine (14% alcohol) and 1-2 ml/kg of 80 proof liquor (40% alcohol). Alcohol is metabolized at about 10-25 mg/dl/hour.

    Symptoms

        Nausea, vomiting, seizures

    Physical Findings

        Stupor, coma, ataxia, nystagmus, apnea

Laboratory Findings
>   Serum ethanol level elevated

Differential Diagnosis
>   Other alcohols

Diagnostic Plan
>   Ethanol level, Chem 18

Therapeutic Plan
>   Not absorbed by activated charcoal
>   Supportive measures, airway/ventilatory support

Prognosis
>   Hemodialysis if serum levels above 450-500 mg/dl

Iron Poisoning

Is now the most common cause of death from ingestion in children (1995).

Etiology
>   Vitamins with iron, including prenatal vitamins and postnatal iron tablets, are common source.

Pathophysiologic Abnormality
>   Ingestion of greater than 50 mg/kg of elemental iron causes toxicity. Iron causes caustic damage to gastrointestinal mucosa and at elevated levels is a mitochondrial poison.

Four Distinct Phases

Phase	Time Period	Mechanism	Manifestation
I	0-6 hours	direct mucosal injury	vomiting, diarrhea, gastrointestinal bleeding
II	2-24 hours	"latent period"	diminished gastrointestinal symptoms
III	24 hours	hepatocellular injury	cyanosis, profound metabolic acidosis
IV	days-weeks	mucosal scarring	pyloric stenosis, intestinal scarring

Potential Complications
>   Phase I: shock, coma
>   Phase III: seizures, coma; intractable shock

Diagnostic Plan
>   Serum iron, iron-binding capacity, CBC, Chem 18, type and cross match blood.

Therapeutic Plan
>   Ipecac if within 30 minutes of ingestion. IV fluids, IV deferoxamine (if serious ingestion), lavage with 1.5% bicarbonate, whole bowel lavage (if iron seen on post-lavage X-ray).

Prognosis
>   Patients with vomiting, diarrhea, serum glucose greater than 150 mg/dl, WBC greater than 15,000/mm^3 and radiopaque material on abdominal X-rays all correlate with serious toxicity risk. Children who are completely asymptomatic 6 hours post-ingestion are not at risk for toxicity.

Organophosphate Poisoning
Etiology
>   Lipid-soluble insecticide found in home and agricultural use.

Pathophysiologic Abnormality
>   Can be absorbed by inhalation, ingestion and through the skin. They irreversibly phosphorylate acetylcholinesterase resulting in accumulation of acetylcholine at cholinergic receptor sites. Symptoms usually develop within 12 hours of a significant exposure.

Symptoms
>   Dizziness, headache, convulsions, ataxia, coma, sweating, tremors, muscle twitching, weakness, paralysis, gastrointestinal cramps, increased urinary frequency, vomiting

Physical Findings
>   Miosis, bradycardia, bronchorrhea, wheezing, lacrimation, acclerated peristalsis

Laboratory Findings
>   Decreased plasma or red blood cell cholinestrase activity is confirmatory but not usually available on stat basis.

Potential Complications
>   Pulmonary edema

Differential Diagnosis
>   Carbamates cause reversible carbamylation of acetylcholinesterase

Diagnostic Plan

Must usually rely on clinical findings and history of exposure

Therapeutic Plan

Remove clothing, wash skin, protect staff from exposure to their skin. Atropine until bronchorrhea abates (may require high doses). Severe posioning is also treated with pralidoxime (2-PAM); avoid aminophylline and phenothiazine because of their effect on acetylcholine. Carbamates respond to atropine but not to prolidoxime.

Tricyclic Antidepressant Poisoning

Pathophysiologic Abnormality

Some symptoms are due to the anticholinergic effect of these agents. The more life-threatening effects are due to alteration of cellular membrane potential, which may result in ventricular tachycardia, hypotension, and torsades de pointes. Seizures and coma may occur in severe overdoses.

Symptoms

Altered sensorium (lethargy, hallucinations, coma), seizures, urinary retention

Physical Findings

Seizure activity, hypotension, ataxia, pupils dilated (but reactive to light).

Laboratory Findings

Ventricular dysrhythmias on EKG, prolonged QRS internal which may progress to complete heart block and asystole.

Diagnositc Plan

Symptomatic patients should be monitored 48 hours. Serum levels are not helpful.

Therapeutic Plan

Gastric lavage, sodium bicarbonate to raise pH to 7.45-7.5, antiarrhythmic therapy with magnesium, lidocaine or phenytoin. NOTE: Quinidine and procanamide should be avoided.

Prognosis

A QRS interval over 0.1 second on the EKG is associated with significant morbidity and mortality.

Jane E Puls

General Considerations

The abuse of children certainly is not unique to this age or to our society. In ancient times infanticide was practiced by both Greeks and Romans. Children have been sexually "used" and physically abused throughout history. However, societies' recognition of child abuse and neglect and some attempt to prevent or treat this malady is fairly recent.

In the USA today there are approximately 3 million reports of suspected abuse annually. About 1/3 of these, 1 million cases, are confirmed as being abuse or neglect on an annual basis. These numbers have been increasing over time and doubtless will continue to increase as our society and our family structure is fragmented and overwhelmed with violence.

Nationally about half of child abuse cases are neglect, approximately 1/4 are physical abuse, slightly less than that are sexual abuse and the remainder of the cases are made up of psychological maltreatment and Munchausen by Proxy Syndrome. Each of these forms of abuse will be discussed individually.

All fifty states and the District of Columbia have mandatory reporting laws. A mandatory reporting law essentially requires that any person who has or should have reasonable suspicion that a child has been injured or neglected must report that suspicion to the appropriate authorities. All reported suspected cases are investigated and cases are then ruled as confirmed, unconfirmed, or uncertain (unable to determine). Physicians who care for children have a particular obligation to be aware of the forms of child abuse, the historical and physical indicators of abuse, the physical findings (or probable lack there of in sexual abuse), the appropriate diagnostic tests, etc, and medical personnel **must** be willing to become involved in the area of child abuse if they are truly going to care for children.

Death from child abuse deserves special mention. Child abuse deaths nationally are on the rise. They now number about 1,300 a year (this number is likely a gross underestimation, but our investigation and reporting is very incomplete). About 40% of child abuse deaths are from neglect and about 60% are from abuse. The single most common cause of child abuse death is head trauma, and blunt trauma to the head plus shaken baby accounts for more than 40% of all child abuse deaths. Of children who die more than 40% are less than one year and approximately 2/3 are less than 3 years of age. More than 90% of all child abuse death victims are less than 5 years of age. The majority of the perpetrators of child abuse deaths are the natural parents and approximately 40% of the families of child abuse death victims have a history of prior involvement with child protective services. Child abuse has now surpassed falls, drownings, and fires as the leading cause of death of children age 1-4. There is very little that the physician can do on the "fix it" end to address child abuse deaths. We must all work to prevent child abuse in all its forms with parent education, early identification of high-risk and abusive situations, etc.

Categories

Munchausen by Proxy Syndrome
Emotional/Psychosocial Maltreatment
Sexual Abuse
Neglect
Physical Abuse

Munchausen by Proxy Syndrome
Alternate Terminology
Munchausen Syndrome by Proxy (the name has been altered from this to make it clear that the disease is the proxys, and not the child's).

Definition
A situation in which a parent of caretaker persistently fabricates information about a child's health or induces illness in a child in order to seek medical attention.

Etiology
Severe, poorly understood psychopathology in the perpetrator (**most often the mother**). Munchausen by Proxy Syndrome is a bizarre form of abuse in which the perpetrator uses a child so that they can establish a relationship with a medical system. Usually one child at a time in a family is the victim, but perpetrators may injure or kill multiple children over the course of their disease. Many people doubt that the perpetrator's illness is "curable", and feel that terminating their contact with children is the only solution.

Presentation
The child with Munchausen by Proxy Syndrome is usually "presented" to the medical system by the mother either with a history of significant medical problems or with actual symptoms of a disease. Perpetrators are generally either "fabricators", individuals who make up medical history about their child or "inducers", individuals who actually injure their child, or give their child medications, infections, poisonings, etc, to create an illness in the child. The parent will repeatedly seek medical attention for the child and generally becomes very involved in the child's medical support system. The medical community generally adds to the child's ills by doing a long evaluation and many diagnostic tests on the child in an

effort to address the child's "illness". It is only when the child repeatedly comes to medical attention but his "disease" does not make sense that the medical community begins to suspect the diagnosis of M by PS. It isn't reasonable to think that medical personnel should suspect every parent who seeks medical attention of creating illness in their child; however, it is critically important that, if a child's history or presentation is not usual or typical the possibility that the child's illness has been fabricated or induced be entertained.

Differential Diagnosis

The differential diagnosis for Munchausen by Proxy Syndrome is true disease in the child. Most illnesses that a child could truly have can be fabricated or induced by a parent or caretaker. Some of the more common presentations of M by PS involve apneic episodes (which may be fabricated or which may actually be induced by the parent, but occur only when the perpetrator is alone with the child), seizures, recurrent vomiting (which may be induced by the administration by Ipecac repeatedly to a child), chronic diarrhea (induced by laxatives), and sepsis (which is sometimes created by injecting children with feces or other contaminated material).

Management

When a child is repeatedly seen for a medical problem that is not reasonable given their circumstances the diagnosis of Munchausen by Proxy Syndrome should be entertained. Once this has occurred all members of the medical system should make note of the circumstances surrounding the child's presentation, do very careful documentation of historical information, complaints, parents behavior, etc. Early identification of the child at risk and removal of the child from the home circumstance is imperative. Once the child's protection is insured then efforts can be begun to resolve the situation. As mentioned previously there is much that is unknown about likely outcome in these situations.

Emotional or Psychological Maltreatment
Definition

Emotional and psychological maltreatment are grouped together. In general emotional maltreatment is a situation in which a child is not provided with appropriate support, attention and affection. Psychological maltreatment is generally considered as a chronic pattern of behavior such as humiliating, ridiculing, or belittling a child. Both of these forms of maltreatment may result in impaired psychological growth and development of the child.

Presentation

Many, many children in our society have inadequate parenting. To define a child as emotionally or psychologically maltreated is very difficult. Certainly we see reflections of some degree of psychological or emotional maltreatment in many of our abused children. Children who have sleep disturbances or sleep disorders, who have encopresis, who have developmental delays, speech disorders, habit disorders, or behavioral extremes should be considered as possibly psychologically or emotionally maltreated.

Differential Diagnosis

Any child who's history or presentation suggest an emotional or psychological problem should have further investigation of their family background, life situation, academic achievement, and personality.

Management

Any physician who truly feels that a child is being emotionally or psychologically maltreated should refer the situation to the juvenile justice system as well as seeking help in the management of the child from appropriate counselors, psychologists, psychiatrists, etc.

Sexual Abuse

Definition

Sexual abuse is generally considered to be sexual activity that involves children, that is inappropriate to the child's developmental level, does not have the child's informed consent and violates societies taboos. Note: As a general rule there is a discrepant age between the child and the perpetrator but we now see many juveniles perpetrating against other children. When we talk about sexual abuse in children we do not talk about sexual play, sexual exploration or other sexual activity that is appropriate to the child. We talk about sexual activity that is inappropriate for that child and **that is done for the sexual gratification of the perpetrator.**

Terminology

When we talk about sexual activities that involve children we talk in specific language about what has happened to the children. It is important to remember that most sexual abuse of children is non-violent, that it does not cause **physical** harm to the child and that it is most definitely not normal non-sexual contact.

- Fondling - touching directly or through the clothes
- Oral sex
- Simulated intercourse - also called vulvar intercourse

- Intercourse
- Sodomy

Incidence

Numbers vary greatly in any given year and from study to study but across all ages our best information indicates that 1 in 4 females and 1 in 6 males will be sexually abused by the time they reach their 18th birthday.

Presentation

Most sexual abuse is non-violent. The vast majority of children who are abused know their assailant. Many of them are molested on a chronic basis in their home environment. For a multitude of reasons, there is a delay in their disclosure of their abuse. Children who have been the victims of sexual abuse present to the medical system in many ways.

Children may have spontaneous disclosure of their abuse to medical personnel or to someone else. **It is important to remember that when children spontaneously disclose abuse in age-appropriate language and with developmentally appropriate historical description that history is almost never fabricated.** Children may not have direct disclosure of sexual abuse but may have inappropriate sexual activity, inappropriate sexual knowledge, have a sexually transmitted disease, or be pregnant.

Many children present with a very indirect indicator of sexual abuse. They may have non-specific genital, urinary or anal complaints (for instance history of frequent UTIs, vaginal discharge, pain, irritation, etc), have recurrent abdominal pain, headaches, dizziness or weakness, chest pain, behavioral changes, eating disorders, school problems, social problems (for instance hyperactivity, sexualized behavior, acting out behavior), or, in the older child, behavioral sequelae of sexual abuse including depression, suicidal gestures, running away, substance abuse, prostitution or sexual promiscuity.

A complete medical and social history is imperative in evaluating the child for sexual abuse. Questions about a history of sexual abuse must be asked without embarrassment, with the knowledge that children frequently feel guilty about what has happened and are likely to blame themselves, with age-appropriate non-leading questions, and with the patience to let a child describe in their own way, in their own time, in their own words, what has happened to them.

The vast majority of physical exams done on children who have been the victims of sexual abuse are normal and it is **critical** that an adequate history be obtained.

Physical Exam

A complete physical exam should be done to insure the child's well-being. A genital examination should be completed and good documentation of exam findings done. It is important to be familiar with the normal anatomy of the pre-pubertal child so that a description of genital anatomy beyond "Tanner Stage I" can be done. In general the physician should "say what you see" on the genital examination of the child. Describe the size, shape and color of the hymen and any scars, synechia, healed lacerations, bruising, etc, that might be present. On males describe the penis and scrotum and the presence or absence of testicles. A general description of the anus on all children is appropriate.

Testing for sexually transmitted diseases is reasonable in many children who are the victims of sexual abuse. At the present time recommendations for STD testing are somewhat vague. The general recommendation is "appropriate" testing be done for an individual child based on their sexual abuse history and known risk factors in the perpetrator. In part STD testing must be governed by the prevalence of certain diseases in the child's locale.

Management

The single most important part of the management of the sexually abused child is the care of the child and our efforts to reassure them that what has happened to them is in no way their fault, that they do not have to continue to live in an abusive situation, that they are medically okay and that they will grow up to medically "normal". Note: Many children who have been sexually abused believe that they are no longer sexually "good", that they will never be able to have children or have a normal sexual relationship with another person. It is our primary role as physicians caring for children to truly "care for" the child.

Any suspicion of sexual abuse should be reported to the appropriate authority, good medical documentation done and whatever court involvement or other social service involvement is appropriate be done.

Any sexually transmitted diseases that are found in the child should be treated and follow up should be done.

All children who have a significant history of sexual abuse should be referred for counseling.

Remember

- Females have persistence of maternal estrogen effect for up to 2 years and may have fimbriated estrogenized hymens until 2 years of age.
- All females with normal genital anatomy are born with a hymen.
- Hymens in the pre-pubertal child without estrogen effect are usually either annular or crescentic in shape and are sensitive to touch.
- Most child sexual abuse is non-violent and the question "Has anyone ever hurt you down there?" is an inadequate attempt to obtain a history of sexual abuse from a child.
- Many sexually promiscuous adolescents got their introduction to sexual activity through sexual abuse.
- A pregnant 12-year-old is sexually abused.
- Partly because there is a delay in disclosure of sexual abuse, any injuries that might have occurred at the time of the abuse are usually resolved by the time we see children.
- Gonorrhea grows well in the oral pharynx, Chlamydia does not.
- A non-traumatic medical exam is critical: children who are sexually abused have **already** been traumatized.
- As a general rule children do not have hemorrhoids and the presence of these in a child should lead one to think about the possibility of sexual abuse.
- Sexually transmitted diseases are **sexually** transmitted and the presence of a STD in a child must be investigated.
- As a general rule children do not lie about sexual abuse. A well-documented history remains the single most important tool in the evaluation of the sexually abused child.

Neglect

Definition

Neglect is generally considered to be the failure of a parent or caretaker to provide a child under the age of 18 with basic needs such as appropriate shelter, food, clothing, etc, with appropriate supervision and protection or with appropriate medical care when the absence of that medical care might endanger the child's life or well-being.

Incidence

Discussed above. Note: The majority of the children in our society who are neglected are undoubtedly not identified. Many children live their whole life in a neglectful, nonsupportive environment because their parents are not able to parent any better than that. Neglect is by far the most common form of child abuse, yet it is estimated that the vast majority of neglected children do not have contact with the medical profession.

Patient Presentation

As with other forms of child abuse the presentation of the neglected child varies greatly, from the child who at a well-child exam is noted to be growing substandard because of inadequate nutritional provision in their home environment to the 6-month-old who presents to the emergency room for resuscitation after having been left unsupervised in the bathtub for 15 minutes. Most cases of child neglect in our society are identified by family, neighbors, family contacts, etc, are evaluated by the child protective services and never actually encounter the medical community. When a child is seen in the medical system and has a history that would suggest a neglectful environment or has evidence of medical neglect, it is important that we identify these children and get them access to social services and support as soon as possible. If children are inadequately clothed, have a history of having inadequate food, shelter, etc, or are growing inadequately for age, the possibility for neglect should be considered. The two areas of neglect where physicians most commonly have input is in growth failure and medical neglect. Those two subjects are briefly discussed individually below.

Growth Deficiency

Historically called failure to thrive, growth deficiency or growth failure is a situation in which a young child fails to follow their growth curve, fails to have adequate increase in height and weight over time or falls across multiple percentile lines on growth charts. The vast majority of growth deficiency is attributable to inadequate nutritional intake by the child, sometimes for a multitude of reasons.

If a child is noted to be growing inadequately information should be gathered about the child's home environment, feeding methods, nutritional intake, etc. Many children who have failed to thrive have parents who truly care about the child but don't have a good understanding of children's nutritional needs and abilities. People attempt to feed their children inappropriate foods for age, expect children to be able to feed themselves early, etc. Infants are frequently fed "on demand" and if a child is undemanding and does not cry to be fed they may not be given adequate nutrition. Children need to be fed in a consistent and positive manner with adequate appropriate foods in a supportive environment in order to grow well. It is frequently difficult to accomplish that in our society.

Medical management of the child who is growing inadequately involves parent education, record keeping about foods consumed, frequent weight checks and close follow up. Occasionally when a child has extreme failure to thrive and the environmental situation warrants, hospitalization is necessary. It is important to remember that children have development of the central nervous system during intrauterine life and the first 18 months of extrauterine life and it is critical that the child be provided adequate nutritional support during this time.

Medical Neglect

Medical neglect is usually discussed in circumstances where a child has a chronic medical disease and the parents fail to provide needed medications or appropriate medical care and follow up. We also occasionally identify medical neglect in situations of acute illness in children where a **reasonable** parent should know to seek medical care and the parents do not.

When a child has a chronic illness and the provision of a certain environment, certain medications, etc, is critical to the child's medical well-being we require that parents or caretakers provide that medication, environment, etc. Their failure to do so is considered medical neglect and necessitates either that the situation or environment be resolved or that the child be removed from their home. This involves a great deal of effort on the part of the medical community to document the child's medical needs, show that the parents are failing to provide for those needs and attempt to provide whatever services are necessary to help the parents in the care of the child.

Physical Abuse

Definition

Physical abuse is generally defined as any nonaccidental injury to a child under the age of 18 by a parent or caretaker. Note: This is injury that occurs for any reason and that involves tissue damage. As a general rule we also include physical discipline in a child younger than 12 months of age as physical abuse. This excludes injury that one child does to another (including adolescent homicides perpetrated by other adolescents).

Incidence

Discussed above.

Patient Presentation

The presentation of the physically abused child varies, from the child with minor bruising on the buttocks as a result of inappropriate discipline to the child who presents in asystole as a result of abusive head injury. Some children disclose physical abuse while others have their physical abuse found incidentally or because a child supervisor is suspicious when a child wears concealing clothing that is inappropriate to the weather or has inappropriate or defensive behavior. Physical abuse occurs in all segments of the population but certain groups are more at risk and sometimes there are clues in the medical history that makes the possibility of physical abuse more likely.

Risk Factors

- Low-income family
- Young parents
- History of substance abuse in the family
- Criminal history in a parent
- Premature birth in the child
- Chronic illness or developmental disorder in the child

Historical Clues

- Discrepant history
- Injury not consistent with age or developmental ability of the child
- Delay in seeking care
- History of using multiple hospitals or clinics
- Crisis situation for the abuser
- Social isolation
- Unwitnessed "accident"
- Inappropriate parental affect
- Prior history of abuse in the home

Physical Examination

Findings on the physically abused child vary and may include bruises, abrasions, scratches, burns, fractures, abdominal injuries, head injury or any combination. It is most critical to remember that the examination of a child requires the removal of their clothing and that any physical injury in a child should be **reasonable** given the child's age and developmental abilities.

Bruises - Note:
- Shapes or imprints
- Location - bony prominence versus soft tissue
- Color of bruises as compared to age of injury
- Geometric or bilateral bruising
- Size of any bite marks

Burns - Note:
- Pattern - glove-like, pantyhose-like, donut shaped, splash burns, burns in diaper distribution
- Severity of physical injury compared to historical information

Visceral Trauma - Note:
- Chest exam with auscultation is imperative
- Examine the abdomen for bowel sounds
- Abdominal exam for tenderness to palpation, evidence of ileus, evidence of bowel obstruction, or any evidence of perforation

Fractures - Note:
- Any fracture in a pre-ambulatory child is concerning
- The vast majority of fractures in children less than 24 months of age are not accidental
- Children less than 24 months of age may accidentally sustain linear skull fractures, toddlers fractures, or have a nurse maid's elbow (radial head dislocation)
- In general spiral fractures in non-ambulatory infants, fractures to the epiphyseal, metaphyseal, physeal region and rib fractures in children less than 2 years of age are considered to be specific for abuse
- In general children less than 2 years of age who have a fracture need a skeletal survey to look for other fractures.

Head Trauma
- Children may have few or no extracranial signs of their injury.
- Retinal hemorrhages may be helpful
- Abusive head trauma is more common in younger children
- The use of MRI or CT is critical (MRI is developing into a much more useful tool)
- Head injury in children may be from shaking or from direct trauma and usually involves shearing or tearing of the vessels with resultant bleeding into the head, cerebral edema and cellular damage intracranially.

Diagnosis
- History
- Physical Exam
- PT/PTT
- Appropriate X-rays
- MRI or CT
- Dating of injuries
- Skeletal survey
- Platelet count
- Photographs (if appropriate)

Management
- Medical management of the patient is dependent on the nature of the child's physical injury.
- Notification of child protection services and protection of the child is ultimately important.
- Eventual involvement with the legal system may be necessary.
- Long-term medical management or medical follow up of the child should be arranged.

Remember
- Most children who are the victims of physical abuse are not the victims of a single episode of abuse. Most live in an environment with a pattern of abusive behavior.
- The average comfort temperature of water is 105° F. Pain threshold is at approximately 115° F. At this temperature it takes 6 hours to cause first degree burns. Children are not stupid: they do not voluntarily stay in water that is hot enough to burn them.
- Recommendation for home hot water settings is not hotter than 140° F.
- Hot liquids are used in the majority of abusive burns to children and generally do not appear as splash burns on the child but rather appear with a patterned distribution.
- A great deal of information can be obtained by looking at bite marks on a child. Bites perpetrated by other small children should be appropriate in size. Bites perpetrated by animals should have the appropriate pattern to tooth placement.
- The fact that the parents behavior are "appropriate" in an office, clinic or emergency room should in no way be reassuring.

- Children who are pre-ambulatory generally should not have physical injuries. Bruising should not take place in a child too small to be mobile without some adequate explanation
  NOTE: Children do not generally bruise themselves on toys in their playpen when they are less than 6 months of age).
- Inflicted burns in children are most common in the toddler age and are very often related to toilet training issues.
- Spiral fractures require a torsional force and generally should not occur in pre-ambulatory children.
- Children who have Osteogenesis Imperfecta most commonly have a strong family history and physical findings that make that diagnosis very clear (blue sclera, fractures at birth, limb deformity, hearing loss).
- The most common injury seen from abusive abdominal trauma is a duodenal hematoma.
- Chip fractures of the metaphyses occur in children because children's ligaments are stronger than their bones and the bones actually shear off in small pieces. These **small** fractures are **huge** in terms of their importance in the diagnosis of child abuse.
- Mongolian spots can be confused with bruises in small children. They are more common in blacks and Asians and occur most commonly on the buttocks, back and shoulders, but can occur on the extremities or face.
- Infants who fall from "normal" heights (changing table, bed, couch, etc) may sustain simple linear parietal skull fractures but should not have intracranial injuries.
- Children who have been victims of physical abuse may not disclose their abuse. Their angry ugly world may be all they have ever known. Any reasonable suspicion of abuse requires an evaluation and protection of the child.
- The single most important thing to remember when evaluating physical injuries in children is that an assessment of the **reasonableness** of the injury based on the child's age and developmental abilities is critical.

SELF-ASSESSMENT EXAMINATION

1. The American Academy of Pediatrics recommends a certain schedule of health supervision visits. The timing of such visits:

   A. Must accommodate an acceptable immunization schedule
   B. Must accommodate appropriate anticipatory guidance
   C. Must take into consideration the cost to the family
   D. All of the above

2. The most important thing to be learned from anthropomorphic measurements at well child visits is:

   A. How long/tall the child is
   B. How big the child's head is
   C. How the child's weight compares with height
   D. How well the child's measurements are following standard growth curves

3. Which of the following would make you suspect developmental delay?

   A. A 1-year-old child does not walk
   B. A 6-month-old child does not sit alone
   C. A 2-month-old child does not fix gaze or follow
   D. A 4-month-old child does not transfer

4. Which of the following would prompt you to do more than routine screening?

   A. Child living with tuberculous parents
   B. Child whose father had a heart attack at age 50
   C. Child fed homogenized milk from age of 1 month
   D. All of the above

5. Critical sources of information about immunization practices include:

   A. The *Redbook* of the American Academy of Pediatrics
   B. The journal *Pediatrics*
   C. *MMWR*
   D. All of the above

6. An HIV-positive child should not be vaccinated with which of the following:

   A. Any live vaccine
   B. Oral polio vaccine
   C. *Haemophilus influenzae* type b (Hib)
   D. Hepatitis A vaccine
   E. Hepatitis B vaccine

7. Which of the following is (are) combinations of vaccines? (Possible multiple answers.)

   A. MMR vaccine
   B. Varicella vaccine
   C. OPV
   D. HB vaccine

8. Which of the following is (are) absolute and permanent contraindications to vaccination? (Possible multiple answers.)

   A. Pregnancy, for all vaccines
   B. Immunosuppression, for all live vaccines
   C. Onset of encephalopathy within 7 days of a dose, for pertussis vaccine
   D. Blood transfusion, for all live vaccines

9. If you know you could get a family to accept/carry out only one of the following safety measures, which one would you emphasize?

   A. Keep guns out of home, or unloaded and locked
   B. Use proper/effectual restraints in cars
   C. Install smoke alarms
   D. Never allow child to swim alone

10. Which of the following statements is (are) false? (Possible multiple answers.)

    A. The average baby approximately triples in weight by 1 year of age
    B. A fontanelle open to palpation at 18 months of age can be caused by only a very few disorders
    C. A child who can't walk well at 14 months of age is not necessarily abnormal
    D. Sexual maturation in girls begins around 14 years of age
    E. The best time to screen for PKU is as soon after birth as possible

11. A young Asian woman came to the county hospital for delivery of her baby. It was noted that at her last prenatal check up she was positive for hepatitis B

antigen. She also states she doesn't ever remember having been jaundiced at any time in her life. A hepatitis B vaccine should be administered to the child at - (Possible multiple answers)

A. Birth
B. 1-month-old
C. 2-months-old
D. 6-months-old
E. 15-18-months-old

12. A 10-month-old child was rushed to the hospital with an anaphylactic response to neomycin. Which vaccines should not be administered? (Possible multiple answers)

A. MMR
B. OPV
C. DTP
D. IVP
E. Hib

13. Most full-term infants will regain their birth weight by:

A. 48 hours
B. 4 days
C. 14 days
D. 30 days

14. You are attending the delivery of a newborn infant. At one minute of life the infant has a heart rate of 60, no respiratory effort, is cyanotic, has poor tone and doesn't respond to suctioning. The infant's apgar is:

A. 0
B. 1
C. 2
D. 3

15. At 5 minutes of life the same infant has been bagged with O_2 and given Narcan, now his heart rate is 120, he is pink and breathing on his own with a strong cry and grimace at suctioning. He is fully flexed. His apgar is:

A. 8
B. 9
C. 7
D. Unable to determine from information given

16. Each of the following statements about breast feeding is true EXCEPT:

    A. Breast feeding can be initiated in the delivery room for healthy, term infants.
    B. Colostrum is provided by the breasts for 2-3 days and is nutritionally complete.
    C. HIV-positive mothers may breast feed, as there is very low likelihood that an infant will contract HIV from breast milk.
    D. Breast feeding is a learned skill for mother and child and is the preferred feeding method in allowable circumstances.

17. Each of the following suggests respiratory distress in the newborn EXCEPT:

    A. Nasal flaring
    B. Respiratory rate of 46
    C. Cyanosis
    D. Persistent cough

18. A 3-hour-old male born at 34 weeks gestation is tachypneic, with grunting and slightly decreased breath sounds. His arterial blood gas would most closely approximate:

    A. pH 7.42 pO_2 42 pCO_2 42
    B. pH 7.42 pO_2 97 pCO_2 42
    C. pH 7.24 pO_2 97 pCO_2 62
    D. pH 7.24 pO_2 42 pCO_2 62

19. A term infant weighed 3.2 kg and was delivered vaginally with forceps assist after 28 hours of labor. She is now one day old and the nurse reports to you at 11 pm that the child has a temperature of 35.9° C and is not feeding well. You elect to:

    A. Have the nurse check the baby again in four hours
    B. Examine the baby and reassure the nurse
    C. Do blood and urine cultures
    D. Do blood, urine and CSF cultures and begin antibiotic therapy

20. A cephalhematoma can be large enough to cause hyperbilirubinemia when the blood begins to break down.

    A. True
    B. False

21. Which of the following developmental changes is of concern?

    A. An 8-year-old female with breast bud development
    B. A 17-year-old female with Tanner Stage V breast and pubic hair who has not yet begun her menses
    C. A 9 1/2-year-old male who has testes > 1.5 cc in volume
    D. A 16-year-old male who has Tanner Stage V pubic hair and testes, scrotum and penis

22. An 18-year-old female comes to your office for evaluation of failure to begin menses. On physical exam, she has Tanner Stage IV breasts and pubic hair. A pelvic exam reveals a vagina without palpable cervix, uterus or ovaries. The most likely diagnosis is:

    A. Turner syndrome
    B. Hypothalamic-pituitary-ovarian axis disturbance
    C. Testicular feminization
    D. XY karyotype with gonadal enzyme deficiency
    E. Kallmann syndrome

23. Which of the following changes do NOT occur in puberty?

    A. Increase in hypothalamic and pituitary sensitivity to estradiol and testosterone
    B. Increased plasma somatomedin-C
    C. Increased insulin secretion
    D. Increased GHRH secretion
    E. Increase in FSH

24. Which of the following is an ABSOLUTE contraindication to oral contraceptive use in adolescents?

    A. Sickle cell disease
    B. Diabetes
    C. Migraine headaches
    D. Follicular ovarian cyst
    E. Hypertension

25. A 17-year-old female is in the clinic for evaluation of lower abdominal pain and fever. Laboratory reveals increased WBC, slight increase in sed rate. On exam there is significant right adnexal tenderness and cervical motion tenderness. What is the most appropriate therapy for this disease?

A. Ceftriaxone IM and Doxycycline for 14 days
B. Erythromycin for 7 days
C. Benzothine penicillin IM
D. Flagyl po x 7 days
E. Ciprofloxacin po x 10 days

26. A 14-year-old female comes to the clinic for evaluation of a breast mass. On exam, you note a single firm discrete 3 cm mass which seems mobile and is noted in the left upper quadrant of the breast. Most likely diagnosis?

    A. Fibrocystic disease
    B. Accessory breast tissue
    C. Fibroadenoma
    D. Malignant tumor
    E. Gynecomastia

27. A 14-year-old male comes to the clinic for evaluation of testicular pain. The pain began abruptly. He has noticed no penile discharge but he is sexually active. On exam, the left testis is swollen and seems higher than the right. The pain is not relieved by scrotal elevation. Most likely diagnosis?

    A. Epididymitis
    B. Testicular tumor with hemorrhage
    C. Hydrocele
    D. Testicular torsion
    E. Varicocele

28. A 7-year-old male wets the bed at least twice a week. Evaluation and management should include all of the following EXCEPT: (Possible Multiple Answers)

    A. Family history to ascertain if the child's father bed-wet
    B. Bladder exercises
    C. DDAVP
    D. System of positive reinforcement
    E. Use of punishment for failure

29. Encopresis is more common in females than males.

    A. True
    B. False

30. Children should only be diagnosed with migraine headaches if they meet specific criteria.

    A. True
    B. False

31. Most children with poor growth have an underlying organic reason.

    A. True
    B. False

32. Children with Attention Deficit Disorder generally have poor self esteem and significant problems conforming with social norms.

    A. True
    B. False

33. Most genetic malformations are due to:

    A. Mutant genes
    B. Polygenic causes
    C. Deletions
    D. Translocations

34. Prenatal α-fetoprotein is likely to be increased in each of the following EXCEPT:

    A. Trisomy 21
    B. Twins
    C. Neural tube defects
    D. Congenital nephrosis

35. A 3-week-old male presents to the emergency room with a history of vomiting. He appears dehydrated and quite ill, with poor capillary refill, cyanosis and scrotal hyperpigmentation. He has a markedly elevated serum potassium and a metabolic acidosis. His disease occurs as:

    A. A sporadic mutation
    B. An autosomal recessive disorder
    C. An autosomal dominant disorder
    D. An X-linked disorder

36. Match the following:

    a. Female preponderance   A. Hyperthyroidism
    b. Weight gain   B. Hypothyroidism
    c. Autoimmune   C. Both
    d. $\uparrow T_4$, $\downarrow$ TSH   D. Neither
    e. Hashimoto's thyroiditis

37. Which of the following physical findings in boys is the earliest indicator that puberty has begun?

    A. Increasing prostate size
    B. Appearance of upper lip hair
    C. Increasing penile size
    D. Increasing testicular size
    E. Appearance of pubic hair

Match the following. Each answer may be used once, more than once, or not at all.

    A. IgA
    B. IgD
    C. IgE
    D. IgG
    E. IgM

38. A component of human milk in lactating females

39. Binds to human mast cells and can potentially trigger anaphylaxis

40. Ability to cross the human placenta

41. Lowest concentration in serum

42. Highest concentration in serum

43. Clinical characteristics of B-cell defects include:

    A. Decreased serum immunoglobulins
    B. Recurrent infections
    C. Growth is usually delayed
    D. Two of the above
    E. All of the above

44. An 8-month-old child is in the care of the state child welfare system, family history is unknown. Medical history includes two prior hospitalizations for pneumonia, three separate episodes of candidiasis, growth failure and intermittent diarrhea throughout life. This child's evaluation should include:

A. IgG anti-HIV
B. IgA anti-HIV
C. CBC with diff.
D. A and C
E. B and C

45. The following may be suggestive of childhood cancer EXCEPT:

A. Sudden unexplained weight gain
B. Prolonged fever
C. Bone pain
D. Petechiae

46. Common neoplasms causing abdominal masses in early childhood include all the following EXCEPT:

A. Wilm's tumor
B. Neuroblastomas
C. Pancreatic cancer

47. In 1990 the survival rate of children with cancer has risen to:

A. 5%
B. 20%
C. 40%
D. 65%

48. The most common solid tumor in children is:

A. Brain tumor
B. Neuroblastoma
C. Wilm's tumor
D. Hepatoma

49. Potential complications of leukemia in children include all the following EXCEPT:

A. Hyperuricemia
B. Thrombocytopenia
C. Dysfunctional WBCs
D. Polycythemia

50. Of the following, the most likely cause for an acute febrile illness, seen chiefly in the summer and characterized by small vesicles and ulcers surrounded by erythema in the soft palate and anterior tonsillar pillars is:

A. Herpetic stomatitis
B. Coxsackie virus group A
C. Streptococcal pharyngitis
D. Vincent's stomatitis
E. Agranulocytic angina

51. A 3-year-old boy has fever, cough, and a sore throat. He has slightly red conjunctivae and moderate erythema of the soft palate and pharynx. Tonsils are reddened and covered with exudate. The anterior cervical lymph nodes are moderately enlarged. Chest is clear. Leukocyte count is 12,000/mm^3 with 60% polymorphonuclear neutrophils, 2% band forms, and 38% lymphocytes. Of the following, the organism LEAST likely to cause this infection is:

A. *Haemophilus influenzae*
B. Adenovirus
C. Beta-hemolytic streptococcus, group A
D. *Corynebacterium diphtheriae*
E. Epstein-Barr virus

52. An 8-year-old boy became febrile and anorectic four days ago, five days after his return from a summer camping trip. Yesterday, a red macular rash appeared on his ankles and wrists. The rash rapidly spread to the entire body, including scalp, palms and soles, and became more purple and papular. There are now many petechiae and the child complains of headache, malaise, and myalgia. The most likely diagnosis is:

A. Rocky Mountain spotted fever
B. Anaphylactoid (Henoch-Schoenlein) purpura
C. Meningococcemia
D. Lyme disease
E. Kawasaki's disease (mucocutaneous lymph node syndrome)

53. A 2-year-old male develops a sudden fever which rises to 106° F and persists for 3 days. The temperature then abruptly drops to normal and the next day a generalized skin rash appears which lasts for only 18 hours. The most likely diagnosis in this case is:

A. Measles (Rubeola)
B. Chicken pox (Varicella)
C. Rocky Mountain spotted fever
D. Roseola infantum (Exanthem Subitum)
E. German measles (Rubella)

54. Of the following signs, which one is NOT characteristic of scarlet fever?

A. Vesicular rash early in course
B. Sandpaper rash
C. Sore throat
D. Strawberry tongue
E. Patient may appear quite ill

55. A 15-month-old child has a rectal temperature of 40.5 ° C, but does not appear to be seriously ill. No specific findings are evident on the physical examination. White blood cell count is 24,000/mm^3. A blood culture is obtained and is reported to be positive. The most likely etiology of the bacteremia is:

A. *Haemophilus influenzae*, type b
B. *Streptococcus pneumoniae*
C. *Meningococcus*
D. *Staphylococcus aureus*
E. *Streptococcus pyogenes*

56. A 5-year-old white male is being treated for asthma in the emergency room. On initial evaluation he was noted to be tachypneic, with loud inspiratory and expiratory wheezes. When you enter the room to reevaluate him, you notice that he is lying quietly and appears tired. On auscultation, you notice that wheezes are barely audible. Which of the following blood gases is most consistent with this picture?

A. pH 7.48   pCO$_2$ 23   pO$_2$ 55
B. pH 7.40   pCO$_2$ 32   pO$_2$ 40
C. pH 7.24   pCO$_2$ 62   pO$_2$ 55
D. pH 7.44   pCO$_2$ 22   pO$_2$ 60
E. pH 7.36   pCO$_2$ 55   pO$_2$ 50

57. Which of the following conditions is NOT associated with infantile apnea?

A. Seizures
B. Choanal atresia
C. Sepsis/shock
D. Asthma
E. Hypocalcemia

58. Aunt Jody, a third year medical student, was eager to visit her newborn nephew. She anxiously waited to hold him in her arms and give him a kiss. During a quick weekend visit and with her trusty *"OK Peds"* in hand, she got her chance. She held the baby over the weekend and kissed him several times. She began to notice that the baby had a "salty taste" and immediately suggested that the baby be tested for:

A. Insulin-dependent diabetes mellitus
B. Trisomy 18
C. Cystic fibrosis
D. Adrenal hyerplasia
E. Duodenal atresia

59. What is the inheritance pattern for this condition?

A. Autosomal recessive
B. Autosomal dominant
C. X-linked recessive

60. Regarding asthma, which of the following is incorrect?

A. Cigarette smoking in the house is a predisposing factor
B. Recurrent wheezing is not a necessary physical finding to the diagnosis of asthma
C. Cromolyn sodium is a commonly used bronchodilator in the treatment of asthma
D. Peak flow meters can be used at home to monitor pulmonary function
E. Prednisone is appropriate oral therapy for active flare-ups of the disease

61. A 15-month-old white female is admitted with acute onset of wheezing, cough and respiratory distress. Which of the following is the most likely diagnosis?

A. Croup

B. Foreign body aspiration

C. Respiratory syncytial virus infection

D. Epiglottitis

E. Bronchopulmonary aspergillosis

62. Which of the following is not a predisposing condition for bronchopulmonary dysplasia (BPD)?

A. Mechanical ventilation

B. Pulmonary infection

C. Male sex

D. Congenital cyanotic heart defect

E. Prematurity

63. A 1-month-old is seen in the emergency room for respiratory distress. On physical examination he is pale and diaphoretic. Examination of the lungs reveals diffuse crackles bilaterally. Abdominal exam shows normal bowel sounds, no abdominal masses or tenderness, but hepatomegaly is noted. Most likely diagnosis?

A. Pneumonia

B. Asthma

C. Sepsis with vascular compromise

D. Viral hepatitis

E. Congestive heart failure

64. A 10-day-old is in congestive heart failure. On physical exam you might expect to find all of the following EXCEPT:

A. Pedal edema

B. Hepatomegaly

C. Cyanosis

D. Diastolic murmur

E. Hyperdynamic precordium

65. For each heart lesion listed, match any association. Each lesion may have one or more than one association.

a. VSD

b. TAPVR

c. PDA

A. Holosystolic murmur

B. Trisomy

C. "Snowman" appearance of heart on X-ray

D. Produces increased pulmonary blood flow

66. The most common form of congenital heart disease is:

A. Coarctation
B. VSD
C. PDA
D. ASD

67. The most common congenital heart disease found in adults is:

A. Coarctation
B. VSD
C. AS
D. ASD

68. A 9-month-old white male was rushed to the emergency department at the teaching hospital. Unfortunately, the child was dead on arrival - there were so many problems. The pathology report list included strawberry tongue, swollen extremities with desquamation, with death attributed to a ruptured coronary artery aneurysm. This disease is more common in: (Possible Multiple Answers)

A. Blacks
B. Males
C. Spring
D. Fall
E. Japanese

69. An 8-year-old is noted to have small shoe size for age and rib notching on chest X-ray. This child's heart disease is associated with:

A. Williams syndrome
B. Noonan syndrome
C. Marfan syndrome
D. Turner syndrome

70. Each of the following might be appropriate in the treatment of an infant with SVT EXCEPT:

A. Vagal maneuvers
B. Adenosine
C. Verapamil
D. Digitalis
E. Cardioversion

71. While doing a 4th year rural rotation you examine a 9-month-old child with diarrhea. As always you also inquire about development, nutrition and family history. You learn that the mother is a strict vegetarian who has been breastfeeding the infant with goat milk supplementation. Before presenting the case you perform a spun Hct and peripheral smear which suggest a macrocytic anemia. Which two of the following diagnoses are most likely?

    A. Hypothyroidism
    B. B_{12} deficiency
    C. Iron deficiency
    D. Chronic blood loss secondary to Salmonella enteritis from unpasteurized goat's milk.
    E. Folate deficiency

72. A 12-year-old presents to your office with complaint of prolonged heavy menstrual bleeding during this, her first menses. You obtain the following tests: PT normal, PTT prolonged, platelet count - normal. What is your diagnosis?

    A. von Willebrand disease
    B. Hemophilia A
    C. Hemophilia B
    D. Spontaneous abortion with coagulopathy
    E. Platelet function abnormality

73. A 10-month-old boy presents with bruising and gingival hemorrhage. Family history is significant for an uncle with a bleeding problem. Lab: prolonged PTT normal PT. What factor is missing?

    A. III
    B. VII
    C. X
    D. XIII
    E. VIII

74. Hypochromic microcytic anemias include all of the following EXCEPT:

    A. Lead poisoning
    B. β-thalassemia
    C. Hereditary spherocytosis
    D. Iron deficiency
    E. α-thalassemia

75. A 4-year-old boy presents to your office with multiple bruises. He has been afebrile and experienced a viral URI 2 weeks ago. Physical exam is normal except for diffuse petechiae and bruising. Lab: Hgb 12.8 gm/dL, WBC 9,200/mm^3, differential 60% neutrophils, 36% lymphocytes, 5% monocytes, platelet count 4,000. What is the most likely diagnosis?

    A. Aplastic anemia
    B. Acute lymphoblastic leukemia (ALL)
    C. Idiopathic thrombocytopenic purpura
    D. Rocky Mountain spotted fever
    E. Meningococcemia

76. A concerned mother brings her 2-year-old to you with questions about his behavior. After a complete history you obtain a venous blood lead level of 40 mcg/dL. What is the MOST likely source of the lead poisoning?

    A. Soil
    B. Household dust in 40-year-old home
    C. Lead-contaminated drinking water from lead pipes
    D. Lead-glazed pottery
    E. Folk remedies

77. During a 12-month-old's well-child visit you obtain a spun Hct of 27%. Further laboratory findings include Hgb 9g/dL, MCV 63, retic count 1.8%. What is the most likely etiology of the iron deficiency anemia in this child?

    A. Lead ingestion
    B. Chronic blood loss
    C. Chronic infections
    D. Iron malabsorption
    E. Inadequate dietary intake

78. An increase in the mean corpuscular hemoglobin concentration suggests:

    A. An increase in the weight of hemoglobin
    B. Spherocytosis
    C. A measure of heterogeneity of RBC sizes
    D. Iron deficiency
    E. Thalassemia

79. All of the following are examples of a macrocytic-normochromic anemia EXCEPT:

   A. B_{12} deficiency
   B. Hypothyroidism
   C. Lead poisoning
   D. Fanconi's anemia
   E. Hypoplastic anemia

80. Which of the following minerals is required for site-specific absorption of vitamin B_{12}?

   A. Calcium
   B. Cobalt
   C. Phosphorus
   D. Potassium
   E. Iron

81. Hirschsprung's disease commonly manifests in the newborn as:

   A. Abdominal mass
   B. Diarrhea
   C. Intestinal obstruction
   D. Sepsis

82. Vomiting in the first two days of life can be caused by all of the following EXCEPT:

   A. Pyloric stenosis
   B. Duodenal atresia
   C. Malrotation of gut
   D. Esophageal atresia

83. All of the following are appropriate current forms of therapy for esophageal reflux EXCEPT:

   A. Prone position
   B. Cisapride
   C. Antacids
   D. Thickened feeds

84. Initial therapy in a child with moderately severe upper gastrointestinal blood loss would include:

   A. Normal saline bolus
   B. Blood replacement
   C. Nasogastric suction
   D. All of the above

85. Match the following disease and therapy:

   a. Primary lactose intolerance   A. Pancreatic enzymes
   b. Inflammatory bowel disease   B. Gluten-free diet
   c. Pancreatic insufficiency   C. Steroids
   d. Celiac disease   D. Lactose supplements

86. Pancreatic insufficiency in childhood is commonly due to:

   A. Autoimmune disease
   B. Biliary atresia
   C. Carcinoma
   D. Cystic fibrosis

87. A decreased serum complement level is NOT expected in which of the following:

   A. Poststreptococcal glomerulonephritis
   B. Idiopathic nephrotic syndrome
   C. Systemic lupus erythematosis
   D. Membranoproliferative glomerulonephritis

88. Indications for dialysis in children do NOT include:

   A. Fluid overload
   B. Metabolic acidosis
   C. Hypokalemia
   D. Coagulation disturbances

89. Which of the following is NOT an expected finding in nephrotic syndrome in children?

   A. Proteinuria
   B. Hyperlipidemia
   C. Hypertension
   D. Edema

90. Uncomplicated poststreptococcal glomerulonephritis in children is characterized by all the following EXCEPT:

    A. Decreased serum complement level
    B. Hypertension
    C. RBC casts in urine
    D. Urine protein loss greater than 100 mg/kg/day

91. Which of the following is NOT characteristic of prerenal oliguria?

    A. BUN/Cr ratio > 20:1
    B. Urine specific gravity > 1.015
    C. Fractional excretion of sodium > 3%

92. The findings of purpuric lesions which are palpable (indurated) in a child rules out the possbility of the child having Henoch-Schönlein purpura.

    A. True
    B. False

93. The normal daily maintenance fluid requirement for a 25 kg child is:

    A. 2500 cc/day
    B. 2100 cc/day
    C. 1600 cc/day
    D. 1000 cc/day

94. Hyponatremia with a normal BUN is NOT seen in which of the following:

    A. Inappropriate ADH secretion
    B. Dehydration due to pyloric stenosis
    C. Water intoxication

95. With adequate treatment of dehydration in a child with normal kidneys, one can expect an elevated BUN to decrease by 1/2 every:

    A. 1-2 hours
    B. 4-8 hours
    C. 15-20 hours
    D. 24-36 hours

96. A 0.1 acute increase in serum pH will generally cause the serum potassium to:

A. Increase 0.5 mEq/l
B. Decrease 0.5 mEq/l
C. Increase 0.1 mEq/l
D. Decrease 0.1 mEq/l
E. Remain unchanged

97. Causes of increased anion gap metabolic acidosis include all the following EXCEPT:

A. Methanol poisoning
B. Lactic acidosis
C. Acute diarrhea with HCO_3 and Cl^- losses
D. Ethylene glycol poisoning
E. Aspirin toxicity

98. Which of the following is NOT a normal cerebral spinal fluid value for a child over 6 months of age?

A. Protein 30 mg/dl
B. Segmented neutrophils 8/mm^3
C. RBCs 3/mm^3
D. Glucose 1/3 of blood glucose

99. Inborn errors of metabolism are a common cause of altered mental status in the adolescent.

A. True
B. False

100. Which of the following is NOT characteristic of an upper motor neuron lesion?

A. Posture: flaccid
B. Reflexes: increased
C. Fasciculations: absent
D. Muscle tone: increased

101. The most common cause of macrocephaly in infants is:

A. Brain tumors
B. Hydrocephalus
C. Lead poisoning
D. Excessive growth hormone

102. Two or more café au lait spots are diagnostic of neurofibromatosis, if they are at least 10 cm in diameter each.

   A. True
   B. False

103. Kayser-Fleischer rings in the cornea is characteristic of:

   A. Tay-Sachs disease
   B. Neimann-Pick disease
   C. Wilson disease
   D. All of the above

104. A 2-year-old black male is brought for evaluation of bowed legs. His mother says that he started walking at approximately nine months of age and she noticed it after that time. She feels the bowing has worsened significantly. On examination you note that the right leg seems more bowed than the left, although leg lengths appear symmetrical. Which of the following therapeutic options is most appropriate?

   A. Follow the child clinically, as most children with "bowlegs" have resolution of the deformity as they grow older.
   B. Send the child to an orthopedic specialist for corrective shoe fitting.
   C. Obtain X-rays of both extremities to look for evidence of Blount's disease.
   D. Obtain X-rays of the hip and pelvis to look for evidence of Legg-Calve-Perthes disease.
   E. Send the child to an orthopedic specialist for surgical correction of the deformity.

105. An 8-month-old black female is brought to the emergency room with prolonged crying and irritability. Mom has noticed no rhinorrhea, fever, cough, vomiting or diarrhea. On examination you notice swelling of her hands and feet which is symmetrical. Her mother has noticed this, a time or two previously, but did not bring her to the doctor. An X-ray of the feet shows radiographic changes with early bony sclerosis. Most likely diagnosis?

   A. Juvenile rheumatoid arthritis
   B. Hemophilia
   C. Sickle cell disease
   D. Charcot-Marie-Tooth disease

106. Which of the following orthopedic deformities do NOT require serial casting or surgical correction?

    A. Pes planus (flatfoot)
    B. Metatarsus varus
    C. Talipes equinovarus
    D. Metatarsus adductus

107. A 3-month-old infant is being evaluated for a fracture of the left femur. Physical examination except for the fracture is remarkable only for a bluish discoloration of the sclera. What is the most likely diagnosis?

    A. Child abuse
    B. Klippel-Feil anomaly
    C. Still's disease
    D. Pathologic fracture secondary to bone malignancy
    E. Osteogenesis Imperfecta

108. Which of the following is UNTRUE concerning rheumatoid arthritis?

    A. Iridocyclitis is of particular concern in pauciarticular arthritis
    B. The treatment of choice for all three forms is oral steroids, in conjunction with nonsteroidal anti-inflammatories.
    C. Polyarticular arthritis is most common around 8 to 10 years of age and frequently involves fingers, spine, ankles and feet.
    D. It is an autoimmune disorder which causes the release of lysosomal enzymes which break down the articular surface of a joint.
    E. Physical therapy should be included in the treatment regimen.

109. A 12-year-old boy is referred to you because of pain and swelling below his right knee. He is active in sports, particularly basketball and skiing. On physical examination, there is point tenderness over the anterior tubercle of his right knee. The most likely diagnosis is:

    A. Patellar dislocation
    B. Osteochondritis dissecans
    C. Tear of the collateral ligament
    D. Osgood-Schlatter disease
    E. Tear of the medial meniscus

110. During the primary survey of trauma victims, treatable causes of inadequate breathing include all of the following EXCEPT:

A. Tension pneumothorax
B. Flail chest
C. Cardiac tamponade
D. Transected trachea
E. All the above are correct

111. Nasogastric tubes are always indicated in patients with facial fractures as part of the initial stabilization process.

A. True
B. False

112. Indications for intubation of the comatose child includes all the following EXCEPT:

A. Inability to maintain patent airway
B. Absent gag reflex
C. Impending brainstem herniation due to increased intracranial pressure
D. Glasgow coma score < 12

113. The Glasgow Coma Score involves assigning a numeric value to each of the following criteria EXCEPT:

A. Eye opening responses
B. Pulse oximetry reading
C. Best motor responses
D. Verbal responses

114. Excessive ingestion of which alcohol does NOT cause an increased anion gap metabolic acidosis:

A. Ethanol
B. Methanol
C. Isopropyl
D. No alcohols cause metabolic acidosis

115. Emesis should be induced in children with ingestions:

   A. Resulting in coma
   B. That have depressed the gag reflex
   C. That are caustic to mucosal tissue
   D. Of any hydrocarbon
   E. None of the above

116. Which of the following toxin-antidote pairs is false?

   A. Acetominophen: N-acetylcystine
   B. Ethylene glycol: ethanol
   C. Methanol: naloxone
   D. Nitrates: methylene blue
   E. None of the above are correct

117. Which of the following is true if acute acetominophen poisoning is NOT successfully treated?

   A. Liver tenderness within 2 hours of ingestion
   B. High fever
   C. Hepatic toxicity
   D. Respiratory arrest within 12 hours

118. Which of the following is true regarding aspirin poisoning?

   A. Aspirin is NOT toxic to children younger than 2 years of age
   B. The respiratory alkalosis phase is relatively prolonged
   C. It may result in either hyperglycemia or hypoglycemia
   D. Use of sodium bicarbonate as part of the treatment is indicated

119. Which of the following is false regarding iron poisoning?

   A. It rarely causes death in children
   B. It may cause profound metabolic acidosis
   C. Children who are completely asymptomatic 6 hours post ingestion are not at risk for toxicity

120. Child abuse is the leading cause of death in children age 1-4.

   A. True
   B. False

121. The perpetrator in Munchausen by Proxy syndrome is most commonly the father.

   A. True
   B. False

122. Most sexual abuse is perpetrated by strangers, and sexual abuse frequently causes physical harm.

   A. True
   B. False

123. All normal females are born with a hymen.

   A. True
   B. False

124. Infants frequently have intracranial injuries as a result of accidental falls.

   A. True
   B. False

125. The most common injury seen from abusive abdominal trauma is a splenic rupture.

   A. True
   B. False

126. Children with Osteogenesis Imperfecta usually have historical and physical clues to their diagnosis.

   A. True
   B. False

ANSWERS TO SELF-ASSESSMENT EXAMINATION

1.	D	p 1
2.	D	p 2
3.	C	p 5
4.	D	pp 7, 8
5.	D	p 9
6.	B	p 11
7.	A and C	p 9
8.	C	p 10
9.	B	p 15
10.	B, D, and E	pp 4, 7
11.	A, B, D	p 12
12.	A, D	p 11
13.	C	p 20
14.	B	p 19
15.	B	p 19
16.	C	p 20
17.	B	p 21
18.	D	p 23
19.	D	p 25
20.	A	p 27
21.	B	p 41
22.	C	p 42
23.	A	p 36
24.	E	p 56
25.	A	p 54
26.	C	p 47
27.	D	p 51
28.	C, E	p 63
29.	B	p 64
30.	A	p 69
31.	B	p 72
32.	A	p 73
33.	B	p 76
34.	A	p 77
35.	B	p 81
36.	a-C, b-B, c-C, d-A, e-B	pp 83-84
37.	D	p 88
38.	A	p 92
39.	C	p 92
40.	D	p 91
41.	C	p 92

42.	D	p 91
43.	D	p 95
44.	E	p 96
45.	A	p 102
46.	C	p 103
47.	D	p 106
48.	A	p 108
49.	D	p 107
50.	B	p 125
51.	A	pp 126-127
52.	A	pp 136-137
53.	D	p 118
54.	A	p 118
55.	B	p 119
56.	C	p 141
57.	D	pp 139, 146
58.	C	p 153
59.	A	p 153
60.	C	pp 155, 156, 157
61.	B	p 157
62.	D	pp 152-153
63.	E	p 139
64.	A	p 162
65.	a-A,B,D, b-C,D, c-B,D	pp 165, 169, 170, 186
66.	B	p 168
67.	D	p 177
68.	B, C, E	p 187
69.	D	pp 169, 183
70.	C	p 192
71.	B and E	pp 204-205
72.	A	pp 224-225
73.	E	pp 223-224
74.	C	pp 210-211
75.	C	p 227
76.	B	p 209
77.	E	p 207
78.	B	pp 210-211
79.	C	pp 207-208
80.	A	p 205
81.	C	p 237
82.	A	p 236
83.	A	p 236
84.	D	p 244